AIR FRYER COOKBOOK:

FRIED FOOD BECOMES HEALTHY AND THIS
COMPLETE 365 RECIPES GUIDE FOR NEWBIES
WILL SHOW YOU HOW, INCLUDING DIABETICS
AND A 31 DAYS MEAL PLAN TO ACHIEVE YOUR
BURN FAT GOALS RIGHT NOW!

KIMBERLY MADISON

TABLE OF CONTENTS

Introduction

An air frying oven is one of the most sought-after appliances because of its versatility and ease of use. The appliance will cook your food by circulating hot air into the cooking chamber. This is the best choice for individuals who are looking for the best fried foods without compromising its quality. In this book we are going to cover a wide array of cooking ways such as instant vortex air fryer oven. This is a 7 in 1 cooking appliance can perform seven functions of cooking without compromising the quality of foods. The air fryer is exceptionally good because it saves nearly 80% of your oil while frying your food. If you want to make French fries you will need very little oil. It is not limited to only the crunchy foods but also it is highly effective in cooking a wide array of foods.

You can roast a chicken, reheat frozen foods, bake muffins, and dehydrate your fruits as well. The microprocessor technology utilized in the appliance makes it the best in cooking because it of the programmed keys. You can easily cook your foods without worrying about the time and temperature settings. Besides, the air fryer is vital because it reduces excess calories that is often associated with weight gain. The appliance is made to ensure that you get high quality foods without adding more calories. The crunchiness of the food from outside and tender inside is what separates it from the rest of the air fryers. We have covered over 80 recipes in this book and you can choose any of the easy to make recipes and enjoy a meal at the comfort of your home.

Instant air fryer is one of the revolutionary kitchen appliances that will help in making your cooking easy and simple. It is a sophisticated and a more mature version of the old traditional fryer and oven. The air fryer principally circulates hot air inside the vortex of the fryer and this is made possible by the vortex fan. This helps in making the cooking process faster and will make your meals by consuming little oil. The instant vortex fryer is a multicooker kitchen appliance that has seven in built programs.

This means that your fryer can act as a multicooker as it fries, bakes, rotisserie, reheat, broiling as well as rehydrating the foods. It is one of the best replacements for the traditional oven and grill, toaster and dehydrator. Besides, since it is compact in size it will save a lot of space in your kitchen. One of the main benefits of the instant vortex air fryer is that its expanded capacity of the f of air frying allows to cook a large quantity of food at once.

Our main objective is to provide all the information about instant vortex air fryer oven to help you make the right choice. Using this book, you will be able to cook tastier, healthier and fast meals within a short time.

Chapter 1. What is An Air Fryer?

Before we move on, you might be wondering what an air fryer is exactly. Having made its debut in 2010, the air fryer is basically a kitchen appliance that fries without oil. Or, if need be, as little oil as possible. It does this by circulating hot air quickly with a built-in fan, a process that builds temperatures high enough to mimic conventional frying. Because of this, air fryers are able to fry food without the hazards of traditional oil frying – such as oil burns or fire damage – and can do it in a more systematic, controlled manner.

Air Fryer Trouble Shooting Tips

★ Food not cooking perfectly: Follow the recipe exactly. Check whether or not you have overcrowded the ingredients. This is the main reason why food might not cook evenly in an air fryer.

★ White smoke: White smoke is usually the result of grease, so make sure that you have added some water to the bottom drawer to prevent the grease from overheating.

★ Black smoke: Black smoke is usually due to burnt food. You need to clean the air fryer after every use. If you do not, then the remaining food particles are burned when you use the appliance again. Turn the machine off and cool it completely. Then check it for burned food.

★ The appliance won't stop: The fan of the air fryer operates at high speed and needs some time to stop. Do not worry, it will stop soon.

Frequently Asked Questions

1. Q: Can I cook different foods in the air fryer?

A: Yes, you can cook different foods in your air fryer. You can use it for cooking different types of foods like casseroles and even desserts.

2. Q: How much food can I put inside?

A: Different air fryers tend to have different capacities. To know how much food you can put in, look for the "max" mark and use it as a guide to filling the basket.

3. Q: Can I add ingredients during the cooking process?

A: Yes, you can. Just open the air fryer and add ingredients. There is no need to change the internal temperature as it will stabilize once you close the air fryer chamber.

4. Q: Can I put aluminum or baking paper at the bottom of the air fryer?

A: Yes, you can use both to line the base of the air fryer. However, make sure that you poke holes so that the hot air can pass through the material and allow the food to cook.

5. Q: Do I need to preheat?

A: Preheating the air fryer can reduce the cooking time. However, if you forgot to preheat, it is still okay. To preheat the air fryer, simply set it to the cooking temperature and set the timer for 5 minutes. Once the timer turns off, place your food in the basket and continue cooking.

Mistakes to Avoid When Using The Air Fryer

Some models of air fryers use a round basket where foods are cooked while other models will have layered racks that fit into a square cooking space, much like a small oven. My recipes can be used for both baskets and racks.

Keep an eye on timing

You'll find that air fryers cook at different temperatures depending on what model you have. This is why it's important to check on foods during the cooking process, so you don't over or undercook them. If you've cut back on quantities in some of my recipes, be sure to cut the cooking time down accordingly. Remember, my hints are just recommendations to guide you as you use your air fryer.

Using oil sprays

Most of my recipes in this book use oil spray – I use PAM. But you can use any brand you want. Or make your own by merely putting olive oil into a small spray bottle. Use a small amount of oil and spray over the basket and trays to prevent food from sticking. Some of my recipes require you to spray the food with oil directly.

Measurement Conversion Table

Chicken	Temp	Time (min.)		Temp	Time (min.)
Breasts, bone in (1.25 lbs.)	370° F	25	Legs, bone in (1.75 lbs.)	380° F	30
Breasts, boneless (4 oz.)	380° F	12	Wings (2 lbs.)	400° F	12
Drumsticks (2.5 lbs.)	370° F	20	Game Hen (halved – 2 lbs.)	390° F	20
Thighs, bone in (2 lbs.)	380 ° F	22	Whole Chicken (6.5 lbs.)	360° F	75
Thighs, boneless (1.5 lbs.)	380° F	18-20	Tenders	360° F	8-10

Beef	Temp	Time (min.)		Temp	Time (min.)
Burger (4 oz.)	370° F	16-20	Meatballs (3-inch)	380°F	10
Filet Mignon (8 oz.)	400° F	18	Ribeye, bone in (1-inch, 8 oz.)	400° F	10-15
Flank Steak (1.5 lbs.)	400° F	12	Sirloin steaks (1-inch, 12 oz.)	400° F	9-14
London Broil (2 lbs.)	400° F	20-28	Beef Eye Round Roast (4 lbs.)	390° F	45-55
Meatballs (1-inch)	380° F	7			

Pork and Lamb	Temp	Time (min.)		Temp	Time (min.)
Loin (2 lbs.)	360° F	55	Bacon (thick cut)	400° F	6-10
Pork Chops, bone in (1-inch, 6.6 oz.)	400° F	12	Sausages	380° F	15
Tenderloin (1 lb.)	370° F	15	Lamb Loin Chops (1-inch thick)	400° F	8-12
Bacon (regular)	400° F	5-7	Rack of lamb (1.5-2 lbs.)	380° F	22

Fish and Seafood	Temp	Time (min.)		Temp	Time (min.)
Calamari (8 oz.)	400°F	4	Tuna steak	400° F	7-10
Fish Fillet (1-inch, 8 oz.)	400° F	10	Scallops	400° F	5-7
Salmon, fillet (6 oz.)	380° F	12	Shrimp	400° F	5
Swordfish steak	400° F	10			

Chapter 2. 31 Days Meal Plan

Days	Breakfast	Mains	Snack	Dessert
1.	Omelette	Orzo Salad	Zucchini Sauté	Tasty Banana Cake
2.	Cheese Sandwich	Fondant Potatoes	Cumin Eggplant Mix	Simple Cheesecake
3.	Olives Bake	Chicken and Celery Stew	Garlic Kale	Bread Pudding
4.	Tasty Granola	Mushroom Pork Chops	Green Beans Sauté	Bread Dough and Amaretto D essert
5.	Breakfast Sausage	Leftover Mashed Potato Pancakes	Herbed Tomatoes	Cinnamon Rolls and Cream Cheese Dip
6.	Turkey Burrito	Classic Corn Bread Dressing	Coriander Potatoes	Pumpkin Pie
7.	Breakfast Calzone	Crispy Pork Medallions	Creamy Green Beans and Tomatoes	Wrapped Pears
8.	Ham Egg Cups	Nemos Beef with Dry Pepper Lactose Free	Buttery Artichokes	Strawberry Donuts
9.	Mustard Green	Lamb with Potatoes	Sweet Potato and	Air Fried Bananas

			Eggplant Mix	
10.	Banana Oats	Veal Blanquette With Peas	Peppers and Tomatoes Mix	Cocoa Cake
11.	French Toast	Beef Stroganoff	Chives Carrots and Onions	Chocolate Cake
12.	Okra and eggs	Meatballs with Tomatoes and Peas	Cilantro Brussels Sprouts	Apple Bread
13.	Cinnamon Pudding	Cevapi	Garlic Beets	Banana Bread
14.	Veggie Frittata	Milanese Chop	Ginger Mushrooms	Mini Lava Cake s
15.	Loada cauliflower	Lemon Chops	Masala Potatoes	Crispy Apple s
16.	Tomatoes and olives	Amatriciana	Mixed Veggie Chips	Tasty Banana Cake
17.	Avocado Toast	Venetian Liver	Sweet Apple and Pear Chips	Simple Cheesecake
18.	Crispy Ham and eggs	Crispy Pork Medallions	Cocoa Banana Chips	Bread Pudding
19.	Egg, Spinach, and Sausage Cups	Italian Lamb Chops	Coriander Roasted Chickpeas	Bread Dough and Amaretto D essert
20.	Spaghetti squash fritters	Simple Basil Tomatoes	Parmesan Zucchini Chips	Cinnamon Rolls and Cream Cheese Dip
21.	Jalapeno Popper	Parm Asparagus	Ranch Garlic	Pumpkin Pie

			Pretzels	
22.	Olives Bake	Spiced Up Butternut Squash	Herby Sweet Potato Chips	Wrapped Pears
23.	Tasty Granola	Hearty Caramelized Baby Carrots	Cumin Tortilla Chips with Guacamole	Strawberry Donuts
24.	Breakfast Sausage	Sweet Potatoes And Broccoli	Oven-Dried Strawberries	Air Fried Bananas
25.	Turkey Burrito	Cauliflower And Broccoli Dish	Chili Cheese Toasts	Cocoa Cake
26.	Breakfast Calzone	Hearty Lemon Green Beans	Zucchini Sauté	Chocolate Cake
27.	Ham Egg Cups	Green Beans	Cumin Eggplant Mix	Apple Bread
28.	Mustard Green Salad	Glazed Mushrooms	Garlic Kale	Banana Bread
29.	Avocado Toast	Herbed Bell Pepper	Green Beans Sauté	Mini Lava Cake s
30.	Mustard Green Salad	Italian Lamb Chops	Herbed Tomatoes	Crispy Apple s
31.	Olives Bake	Simple Basil Tomatoes	Coriander Potatoes	Tasty Banana Cake

Chapter 3. 365 RECIPES

BREAKFAST RECIPES

Salsa Eggs

Preparation Time: 5 minutes

Cooking time: 20 minutes

Servings: 2

Ingredients:

- ½ green bell pepper, chopped

- ½ red bell pepper, chopped

- 2 eggs, whisked

- 1 tablespoon mild salsa

- Cooking spray

- ½ tablespoon chives, chopped

- Salt and black pepper, to taste

- ¼ cup cheddar cheese, grated

Directions:

1. Grease 2 ramekins with cooking spray and divide the bell peppers into each.

2. In a bowl, mix the eggs with the salsa, chives, salt, and pepper and whisk well.

3. Divide the egg mixture between each ramekin and sprinkle the cheese on top.

4. Preheat the air fryer at 360F. Arrange the ramekins in the frying basket.

5. Cook for 20 minutes at 360F.

6. Serve.

Nutrition:

- Calories: 142

- Fat: 9.4g

- Carb: 5.4g

- Protein: 9.8g

Banana Oats

Preparation Time: 5 minutes

Cooking time: 20 minutes

Servings: 2

Ingredients:

- 1 cup old fashioned oats

- ½ teaspoon baking powder

- 2 tablespoons sugar

- ½ teaspoon vanilla extract

- 1 banana, peeled and mashed

- ½ cup milk

- ½ cup heavy cream

- 1 egg, whisked

- 1 tablespoon butter

- Cooking spray

Directions:

1. In a bowl, mix the oats with the baking powder, sugar, and other ingredients except for the cooking spray and whisk well. Divide the mixture into 2 ramekins.

2. Grease the air fryer with cooking spray and preheat at 340F.

3. Place the ramekins in the air fryer and cook for 20 minutes.

4. Serve.

Nutrition:

- Calories: 533

- Fat: 25.8g

- Carb: 57.9g

- Protein: 11.5g

Jalapeno Popper Egg Cups

Preparation Time: 10 minutes

Cooking time: 10 minutes

Servings: 2

Ingredients:

- 4 eggs
- ¼ cup pickled jalapenos, chopped
- 2 ounces full-fat cream cheese
- ½ cup shredded sharp cheddar cheese

Directions:

1. Beat the eggs in a bowl, then pour into four silicon muffin cups.
2. In a bowl, add cream cheese, jalapenos, and cheddar. Microwave for 30 seconds and stir.
3. Take about ¼ of the mixture and place it in the center of one egg cup.
4. Repeat with the remaining mixture.
5. Place egg cups into the air fryer basket.
6. Cook at 320F for 10 minutes.
7. Serve.

Nutrition:

- Calories: 354
- Fat: 25.3g
- Carb: 2g
- Protein: 21g

CHEESE SANDWICH

Preparation Time: 5 minutes

Cooking time: 8 minutes

Servings: 2

Ingredients:

- 4 cheddar cheese slices

- 4 teaspoons butter

- 4 bread slices

Directions:

1. Place 2 cheese slices between the 2 bread slices and spread the butter on the outside of both pieces of bread.

2. Repeat to assemble the remaining sandwich.

3. Place sandwiches in the air fryer basket and cook at 370F for 8 minutes. Turn halfway through.

4. Serve.

Nutrition:

- Calories: 341

- Fat: 26.8g

- Carb: 9.8g

- Protein 5g

Breakfast Frittata

Preparation Time: 5 minutes

Cooking time: 15 minutes

Servings: 2

Ingredients:

- 1 cup egg whites

- 2 tablespoons chives, chopped

- ¼ cup mushrooms, sliced

- ¼ cup tomato, chopped

- 2 tablespoons milk

- Salt and pepper, to taste

Directions:

1. Preheat the air fryer at 320F.

2. Whisk everything together in a bowl.

3. Spray the frying pan with cooking spray.

4. Transfer frittata mixture to the pan and place it in the air fryer basket.

5. Bake for 15 minutes.

6. Serve.

Nutrition:

- Calories: 78 Fat: 0.6g Carb: 3g Protein: 14.3g

French Toast

Preparation Time: 5 minutes

Cooking time: 6 minutes

Servings: 2

Ingredients:

- 4 bread slices
- 1 tablespoon powdered cinnamon
- 1 teaspoon vanilla extract
- ⅔ cup milk
- 2 eggs

Directions:

1. In a bowl, combine eggs, vanilla, cinnamon, and milk. Mix well.

2. Dip each bread slice into the egg mixture and shake off excess.

3. Place bread slices in a pan.

4. Place pan in the air fryer and cook at 320F for 3 minutes. Flip and cook for 3 more minutes, then serve.

Nutrition:

- Calories: 166 Fat: 6.7g
- Carb: 16.5g Protein: 9.7g

Breakfast Sausage Frittata

Preparation Time: 10 minutes

Cooking time: 10 minutes

Servings: 2

Ingredients:

- 2 eggs

- 1 tablespoon butter, melted

- 2 tablespoons cheddar cheese

- 1 bell pepper, chopped

- 1 tablespoon spring onions, chopped

- 1 breakfast sausage patty, chopped

- Salt and pepper, to taste

Directions:

1. Spray a 4-inch mini pan with cooking spray and set aside.

2. Add chopped sausage patty to a Preparation Timeared dish and air fry at 350F for 5 minutes.

3. Meanwhile, in a bowl, whisk the eggs, pepper, and salt.

4. Add bell peppers, spring onions, and mix well.

5. Once the sausage is done, add them to the egg mixture and mix well, then pour the mixture into the 4-inch pan.

6. Sprinkle with cheese and air fry at 350F for 5 minutes.

7. Serve.

Nutrition:

- Calories: 206

- Fat: 14.7g

- Carb: 6.7g

- Protein: 12.8g

Scrambled Eggs with Toasted Bread

Preparation Time: 5 minutes

Cooking time: 9 minutes

Servings: 2

Ingredients:

- 4 eggs

- 2 bread slices

- Salt and pepper, to taste

Directions:

1. Warm bread slices in the air fryer at 400F for 3 minutes.

2. Add eggs t a pan and season with salt and pepper. Mix well.

3. Place pan in the air fryer and cook at 360F for 2 minutes. Stir quickly and cook for 4 more minutes.

4. Stir well and transfer the scrambled eggs over the toasted bread slices.

5. Serve.

Nutrition:

- Calories: 150

- Fat: 9.1g

- Carb: 5.2g

- Protein: 11.8g

Egg, Spinach, and Sausage Cups

Preparation Time: 5 minutes

Cooking time: 10 minutes

Servings: 2

Ingredients:

- ¼ cup eggs, beaten

- 4 teaspoons shredded jack cheese

- 4 tablespoons spinach, chopped

- 4 tablespoons sausage, cooked and crumbled

- Salt and pepper

Directions:

1. Whisk everything together in a bowl and mix well.

2. Pour batter into muffin cups and place them in the air fryer basket.

3.Bake at 330F for 10 minutes.

4.Cool and serve.

Nutrition:

- Calories: 89

- Fat: 6.3g

- Carb: 1g

- Protein: 7g

Turkey Burrito

Preparation Time: 10 minutes

Cooking time: 10 minutes

Servings: 2

Ingredients:

- 4 slices turkey breast, cooked

- ½ red bell pepper, sliced

- 2 eggs

- 1 small avocado, peeled, pitted, and sliced

- 2 tablespoons salsa

- Salt and black pepper, to taste

- ⅛ cup mozzarella cheese, grated

- Tortillas for serving

Directions:

1. In a bowl, whisk the eggs with salt and pepper. Pour them in a pan and place in the air fryer's basket.

2. Cook at 400F for 5 minutes. Remove from the fryer and transfer eggs to a plate.

3. Arrange tortillas on a working surface. Divide eggs, turkey meat, bell pepper, cheese, salsa, and avocado between them.

4. Roll the burritos. Line the air fryer basket with tin foil and place the burritos inside.

5. Heat up the burritos at 300F for 3 minutes.

6. Serve.

Nutrition:

- Calories: 349

- Fat: 23g

- Carb: 20g

- Protein: 21g

Breakfast Bread Pudding

Preparation Time: 10 minutes

Cooking time: 22 minutes

Servings: 2

Ingredients:

- ¼ pound white bread, cubed
- 6 tablespoons milk
- 6 tablespoons water
- 1 teaspoon cornstarch
- ¼ cup apple, peeled, cored, and chopped
- 2 ½ tablespoons honey
- ½ teaspoon vanilla extract
- 1 teaspoon cinnamon powder
- ¾ cup flour
- ⅓ cup brown sugar
- 1 ½ ounces soft butter

Directions:

1. In a bowl, combine bread, apple, cornstarch, vanilla, cinnamon, honey, milk, and water. Whisk well.

2. In another bowl, combine butter, sugar, and flour and mix well.

3. Press half of the crumble mixture into the bottom of the air fryer, add bread and apple mixture, then add the rest of the crumble. Cook at 350F for 22 minutes.

4. Divide bread pudding onto plates and serve.

Nutrition:

- Calories: 261

- Fat: 7g

- Carb: 8g

- Protein: 5g

Eggs in Avocado Boats

Preparation Time: 5 minutes

Cooking time: 6 minutes

Servings: 2

Ingredients:

- 1 large avocado, cut in half lengthwise

- 2 eggs

- Salt and pepper, to taste

- 1 cup cheddar, shredded

- 1 teaspoon parsley

Directions:

1. Preheat the air fryer at 300F.

2. In a bowl, crack the eggs and mix with the pulp of avocado after de-seeding it.

3. Add salt, pepper, and shredded cheddar.

4. Pour the mixture into the empty avocado halves.

5. Cook in the air fryer for 5 minutes.

6. Sprinkle with chopped parsley and serve.

Nutrition:

- Calories: 450

- Fat: 35g

- Carb: 6g

- Protein: 25g

Ham Egg Cups

Preparation Time: 5 minutes

Cooking time: 12 minutes

Servings: 2

Ingredients:

- 4 (1-ounce) slices deli ham

- 4 eggs

- 2 tablespoons full-fat sour cream

- ¼ cup green bell pepper, diced

- 2 tablespoons red bell pepper, diced

- 2 tablespoons white onion, diced

- ½ cup shredded cheddar cheese

Directions:

1. Place 1 slice of ham on the bottom of 4 baking cups.

2. In a bowl, whisk eggs with sour cream. Stir in onion, red pepper, and green pepper.

3. Pour the egg mixture into the baking cups.

4. Top with cheddar and place cups into the air fryer basket.

5. Cook to 320F for 12 minutes.

6. Serve.

Nutrition:

- Calories: 382

- Fat: 23.6g

- Carb: 4.6g

- Protein: 29.4g

Breakfast Calzone

Preparation Time: 15 minutes

Cooking time: 15 minutes

Servings: 2

Ingredients:

- ¾ cup shredded mozzarella cheese
- ¼ cup almond flour
- ½ ounce full-fat cream cheese
- 1 whole egg
- 2 eggs, scrambled
- ¼ pound breakfast sausage, cooked and crumbled
- 4 tablespoons shredded cheddar cheese

Directions:

1. Add almond flour, mozzarella, and cream cheese to a bowl. Microwave for 1 minute.

2. Stir until the mixture is smooth and forms a ball. Add the egg and stir until dough forms.

3. Place the dough between two sheets of parchment and roll out to a ¼-inch thickness.

4. Cut the dough into four rectangles.

5. In a bowl, mix cooked sausage and scrambled eggs.

6. Divide the blend between each piece of dough, placing it on the lower half of the rectangle. Sprinkle each with cheddar.

7.Fold to cover and seal the edges. Cover the air fryer basket with parchment paper and cook at 380F for 15 minutes. Flip the calzones halfway through the cooking time.

8.Serve.

Nutrition:

- Calories: 560

- Fat: 41.7g

- Carb: 4.2g

- Protein: 34.5g

Omelette

Preparation Time: 5 minutes

Cooking time: 10 minutes

Servings: 2

Ingredients:

- 4 eggs

- ½ cup milk

- Salt, to taste

- Diced fresh meat and veggies – ½ cup (mushrooms, ham, green onions, red bell pepper, etc.)

- 1 teaspoon breakfast seasoning

- ½ cup shredded cheese (mozzarella or cheddar)

- Green onions, for garnish

Directions:

1. Mix the milk and eggs in a bowl until well combined. Season with salt.

2. Add the meat and vegetables to the egg mixture.

3. Pour the mixture into a greased pan. Place the pan into the air fryer basket.

4. Cook 10 minutes at 350F. Around the 5-minute mark, sprinkle the mixture with seasoning and cheese. Finish cooking.

5. Remove from the basket, garnish with green onions, and serve.

Nutrition:

- Calories: 303

- Fat: 19.9g

- Carb: 9.3g

- Protein: 23.1g

Olives bake

Preparation time: 25 minutes

Cooking Time: 15 minutes

servings: 4

Ingredients:

- ½ cup cheddar; shredded

- 4 eggs; whisked

- 2 cups black olives, pitted and chopped.

- 1 tbsp. Cilantro; chopped.

- ¼ tsp. Sweet paprika

- A pinch of salt and black pepper

- Cooking

spray Directions:

Take a bowl and mix the eggs with the olives and all the ingredients except the cooking spray and stir well.

Heat up your air fryer at 350°f, grease it with cooking spray, pour the olives and eggs mixture, spread and cook for 20 minutes. Divide between plates and serve

Nutrition:

calories: 240; fat: 14g;

fiber: 3g; carbs: 5g; protein: 8g

Mustard greens salad

Preparation time: 20 minutes

Cooking Time: 15 minutes

servings: 4

Ingredients:

- ½ lb. Cherry tomatoes; cubed

- 2 cups mustard greens

- 2 tbsp. Chives; chopped.

- 1 tsp. Olive oil

- A pinch of salt and black

pepper Directions:

Heat up your air fryer with the oil at 360°f, add all the ingredients, toss, cook for 15 minutes shaking halfway, divide into bowls and serve for breakfast

Nutrition:

calories: 224;

fat: 8g;

fiber: 2g;

carbs: 3g;

protein: 7g

Cauliflower coconut pudding

Preparation time: 25 minutes

Cooking Time: 20 minutes

servings: 4

Ingredients:

- 3 cups coconut milk

- ½ cup coconut; shredded

- 1 cup cauliflower rice

- 2 tbsp. Stevia

Directions:

In a pan that fits the air fryer, combine all the ingredients and whisk well.

Introduce the in your air fryer and cook at 360°f for 20 minutes

Divide into bowls and serve for breakfast.

Nutrition: calories: 211; fat: 11g; fiber: 3g; carbs: 4g; protein: 8g

Minty eggs

Preparation time: 13 minutes

servings: 4

Ingredients:

1 ½ cup coconut cream

8 eggs; whisked

½ cup mint; chopped.

1 tbsp. Olive oil

Salt and black pepper to taste.

Directions:

Take a bowl and mix the cream with salt, pepper, eggs and mint, whisk, pour into the air fryer greased with the oil, spread, cook at 350°f for 8 minutes, divide between plates and serve

Nutrition:

calories: 212;

fat: 9g; f

iber: 4g;

carbs: 5g;

protein: 11g

Bell pepper eggs

Preparation time: 25 minutes

Cooking Time: 15 minutes

servings: 4

Ingredients:

- 4 medium green bell peppers
- ¼ medium onion; peeled and chopped
- 3 oz. Cooked ham; chopped
- 8 large eggs.
- 1 cup mild cheddar cheese

Directions:

Cut the tops off each bell pepper. Remove the seeds and the white membranes with a small knife. Place ham and onion into each pepper

Crack 2 eggs into each pepper. Top with ¼ cup cheese per pepper. Place into the air fryer basket

Adjust the temperature to 390 degrees f and set the timer for 15 minutes. When fully cooked, peppers will be tender and eggs will be firm. Serve immediately.

Nutrition:

calories: 314;

protein: 24.9g;

fiber: 1.7g;

fat: 18.6g;

carbs: 6.3g

Loaded cauliflower bake

Preparation time: 35 minutes

Cooking Time: 15 minutes

servings: 4

Ingredients:

- 2 scallions, sliced on the bias

- 12 slices sugar-free bacon; cooked and crumbled

- 1 cup shredded medium cheddar cheese.

- 1 medium avocado; peeled and pitted

- ¼ cup heavy whipping cream.

- 1 ½ cups chopped cauliflower

- 6 large eggs.

- 8 tbsp. Full-fat sour cream.

Directions:

Take a medium bowl, whisk eggs and cream together. Pour into a 4-cup round baking dish.

Add cauliflower and mix, then top with cheddar

Place dish into the air fryer basket. Adjust the temperature to 320 degrees f and set the timer for 20 minutes.

When completely cooked, eggs will be firm and cheese will be browned. Slice into four pieces

Slice avocado and divide evenly among pieces. Top each piece with 2 tbsp. Sour cream, sliced scallions and crumbled bacon.

Nutrition: calories: 512; protein: 27.1g;

fiber: 3.2g; fat: 38.3g; carbs: 7.5g

Tasty granola

Preparation time: 15 minutes

Cooking Time: 15 minutes

servings: 6

Ingredients:

- 2 cups pecans; chopped.

- ¼ cup golden flaxseed.

- ¼ cup low-carb, sugar-free chocolate chips.

- 1 cup almond slivers.

- ⅓ cup sunflower seeds.

- ¼ cup granular erythritol.

- 1 cup unsweetened coconut flakes.

- 2 tbsp. Unsalted butter.

- 1 tsp. Ground cinnamon.

Directions:

Take a large bowl, mix all ingredients.

Place the mixture into a 4-cup round baking dish. Place dish into the air fryer basket

Adjust the temperature to 320 degrees f and set the timer for 5 minutes. Allow to cool completely before serving.

Nutrition: calories: 617;

protein: 10.9g; fiber: 11.2g; carbs: 6.5g

Fennel frittata

Preparation time: 20 minutes

Cooking Time: 20 minutes

servings: 6

Ingredients:

- 1 fennel bulb; shredded

- 6 eggs; whisked

- 2 tsp. Cilantro; chopped.

- 1 tsp. Sweet paprika

- Cooking spray

A pinch of salt and black pepper

Directions:

Take a bowl and mix all the ingredients except the cooking spray and stir well.

Grease a baking pan with the cooking spray, pour the frittata mix and spread well

Put the pan in the air fryer and cook at 370°f for 15 minutes. Divide between plates and serve them for breakfast.

Nutrition: calories: 200; fat: 12g;

fiber: 1g; carbs: 5g; protein: 8g

Veggie frittata

Preparation time: 17 minutes

Cooking Time: 15 minutes

servings: 4

Ingredients:

- 6 large eggs.

- ¼ cup chopped yellow onion.

- ¼ cup chopped green bell pepper.

- ½ cup chopped broccoli.

- ¼ cup heavy whipping cream.

Directions:

Take a large bowl, whisk eggs and heavy whipping cream. Mix in broccoli, onion and bell pepper.

Pour into a 6-inch round oven-safe baking dish. Place baking dish into the air fryer basket. Adjust the temperature to 350 degrees f and set the timer for 12 minutes

Eggs should be firm and cooked fully when the frittata is done. Serve warm.

Nutrition:

calories: 168;

protein: 10.2g;

fiber: 0.6g;

fat: 11.8g;

carbs: 3.1g

Avocado cauliflower toast

Preparation time: 23 minutes

Cooking Time: 15 minutes

servings: 2

Ingredients:

- 1 (12-oz.steamer bag cauliflower

- ½ cup shredded mozzarella cheese

- 1 large egg.

- 1 ripe medium avocado

- ½ tsp. Garlic powder.

- ¼ tsp. Ground black pepper

Directions:

Cook cauliflower according to package instructions. Remove from bag and place into cheesecloth or clean towel to remove excess moisture.

Place cauliflower into a large bowl and mix in egg and mozzarella. Cut a piece of parchment to fit your air fryer basket

Separate the cauliflower mixture into two and place it on the parchment in two mounds. Press out the cauliflower mounds into a ¼-inch-thick rectangle. Place the parchment into the air fryer basket.

Adjust the temperature to 400 degrees f and set the timer for 8 minutes

Flip the cauliflower halfway through the cooking time

When the timer beeps, remove the parchment and allow the cauliflower to cool 5 minutes.

Cut open the avocado and remove the pit. Scoop out the inside, place it in a medium bowl and mash it with garlic powder and pepper. Spread onto the cauliflower.

Nutrition:

calories: 278;

protein: 14.1g;

fiber: 8.2g;

fat: 15.6g;

carbs: 15.9g

Okra and eggs

Preparation time: 25 minutes

Cooking Time: 10 minutes

servings: 4

Ingredients:

- 4 eggs; whisked

- 2 cups okra

- 1 tbsp. Butter; melted

- A pinch of salt and black pepper

Directions:

Grease a pan that fits the air fryer with the butter.

In a bowl, combine the okra with eggs, salt and pepper, whisk and pour into the pan

Introduce the pan in the air fryer and cook at 350°f for 20 minutes. Divide the mix between plates and serve.

Nutrition:

calories: 220;

fat: 12g;

fiber: 4g;

carbs: 5g;

protein: 8g

Cinnamon pudding

Preparation time: 16 minutes

Cooking Time: 15 minutes

servings: 2

Ingredients:

- 4 eggs; whisked
- 4 tbsp. Erythritol
- 2 tbsp. Heavy cream
- ½ tsp. Cinnamon powder
- ¼ tsp. Allspice, ground
- Cooking spray

Directions:

Take a bowl and mix all the ingredients except the cooking spray, whisk well and pour into a ramekin greased with cooking spray

Add the basket to your air fryer, put the ramekin inside and cook at 400°f for 12 minutes. Divide into bowls and serve for breakfast.

Nutrition:

calories: 201;

fat: 11g; fiber: 2g; carbs: 4g; protein: 6g

Tomatoes and olives eggs

Preparation time: 20 minutes

Cooking Time: 15 minutes

servings: 4

Ingredients:

- 1 cup kalamata olives, pitted and sliced

- 4 eggs; whisked

- 1 cup cherry tomatoes; cubed

- A pinch of salt and black pepper

- Cooking spray

Directions:

Grease the air fryer with cooking spray, add all the ingredients, toss, cover and cook at 365°f for 10 minutes.

Divide between plates and serve for breakfast

Nutrition:

calories: 182;0

fat: 6g;

fiber: 2g;

carbs: 4g;

protein: 8g

Spaghetti squash fritters

Preparation time: 23 minutes

Cooking Time: 20 minutes

servings: 4

Ingredients:

- 2 cups cooked spaghetti squash

- 2 stalks green onion, sliced

- 1 large egg.

- ¼ cup blanched finely ground almond flour.

- 2 tbsp. Unsalted butter; softened.

- ½ tsp. Garlic powder.

- 1 tsp. Dried parsley.

Directions:

Remove excess moisture from the squash using a cheesecloth or kitchen towel.

Mix all ingredients in a large bowl. Form into four patties

Cut a piece of parchment to fit your air fryer basket. Place each patty on the parchment and place into the air fryer basket

Adjust the temperature to 400 degrees f and set the timer for 8 minutes. Flip the patties halfway through the cooking time. Serve warm.

Nutrition: calories: 131; protein: 3.8g; fiber: 2.0g; fat: 10.1g; carbs: 7.1g

Crispy ham egg cups

Preparation time: 17 minutes

Cooking Time: 15 minutes

Servings: 2

Ingredients:

- 4 large eggs.

- 4 (1-oz.slices deli ham

- ½ cup shredded medium cheddar cheese.

- ¼ cup diced green bell pepper.

- 2 tbsp. Diced red bell pepper.

- 2 tbsp. Diced white onion.

- 2 tbsp. Full-fat sour cream.

Directions:

Place one slice of ham on the bottom of four baking cups.

Take a large bowl, whisk eggs with sour cream. Stir in green pepper, red pepper and onion

Pour the egg mixture into ham-lined baking cups. Top with cheddar. Place cups into the air fryer basket. Adjust the temperature to 320 degrees f and set the timer for 12 minutes or until the tops are browned. Serve warm.

Nutrition: calories: 382; protein: 29.4g; fiber: 1.4g; fat: 23.6g; carbs: 6.0g

LUNCH RECIPES

Monkey Salad

Preparation Time: 5 minutes

Cooking Time: 10 minutes

Servings: 1

Ingredients

★ 2 tbsp butter

★ 1 cup unsweetened coconut flakes

★ 1 cup raw, unsalted cashews

★ 1 cup raw, unsalted s

★ 1 cup 90% dark chocolate

shavings Directions

1. In a skillet, melt the butter on a medium heat.

2. Add the coconut flakes and sauté until lightly browned for 4 minutes.

3. Add the cashews and s and sauté for 3 minutes. Remove from the heat and sprinkle with dark chocolate shavings.

4. Serve!

Nutrition:

calories 270,

fat 15, fiber 3, carbs 5, protein 9

Jarlsberg Lunch Omelet

Preparation Time: 5 minutes

Cooking Time: 10 minutes

Servings: 2

Ingredients

- 4 medium mushrooms, sliced, 2 oz

- 1 green onion, sliced

- 2 eggs, beaten

- 1 oz Jarlsberg or Swiss cheese, shredded

- 1 oz ham,

diced Directions

1.In a skillet, cook the mushrooms and green onion until tender.

2.Add the eggs and mix well.

3.Sprinkle with salt and top with the mushroom mixture, cheese and the ham.

4.When the egg is set, fold the plain side of the omelet on the filled side.

5.Turn off the heat and let it stand until the cheese has melted.

6.Serve!

Nutrition:

Calories: 96

Fat: 8.8g Carbohydrates: 5.12g Protein: 1.2g Sugar: 0.4g Cholesterol: 0mg

Mu Shu Lunch Pork

Preparation Time: 5 minutes

Cooking Time: 10 minutes

Servings: 2

Ingredients

- ★ 4 cups coleslaw mix, with carrots

- ★ 1 small onion, sliced thin

- ★ 1 lb cooked roast pork, cut into ½" cubes

- ★ 2 tbsp hoisin sauce

- ★ 2 tbsp soy

sauce Directions

1. In a large skillet, heat the oil on a high heat.

2. Stir-fry the cabbage and onion for 4 minutes until tender.

3. Add the pork, hoisin and soy sauce.

4. Cook until browned.

5. Enjoy!

Nutrition: 398

Calories; 21g

Fat; 4.7g

Carbs; 44.2g Protein; 0 .5g Sugars

Fiery Jalapeno Poppers

Preparation Time: 10 minutes

Cooking Time: 40 minutes

Servings: 4

Ingredients

- ★ 5 oz cream cheese

- ★ ¼ cup mozzarella cheese

- ★ 8 medium jalapeno peppers

- ★ ½ tsp Mrs. Dash Table Blend

- ★ 8 slices

bacon Directions

1. Preheat your fryer to 400°F/200°C.

2. Cut the jalapenos in half.

3. Use a spoon to scrape out the insides of the peppers.

4. In a bowl, add together the cream cheese, mozzarella cheese and spices of your choice.

5. Pack the cream cheese mixture into the jalapenos and place the peppers on top.

6. Wrap each pepper in 1 slice of bacon, starting from the bottom and working up.

7. Bake for 30 minutes. Broil for an additional 3 minutes. Serve!

Nutrition: Calories: 156 Fat: 8.01g Carbohydrate: 20.33g Protein: 1.98g Sugar: 0.33g

Cholesterol: 0mg

Bacon & Chicken Patties

Preparation Time 5 minutes

Cooking Time: 15 minutes

Servings: 2

Ingredients

- ★ 1 ½ oz can chicken breast

- ★ 4 slices bacon

- ★ ¼ cup parmesan cheese

- ★ 1 large egg

- ★ 3 tbsp

flour Directions

1. Cook the bacon until crispy.

2. Chop the chicken and bacon together in a food processor until fine.

3. Add in the parmesan, egg, flour and mix.

4. Make the patties by hand and fry on a medium heat in a pan with some oil.

5. Once browned, flip over, continue cooking, and lie them to drain.

6. Serve!

Nutrition: Calories: 156 Fat: 8.01g Carbohydrate: 20.33g

Protein: 1.98g Sugar: 0.33g

Cholesterol: 0mg

Cheddar Bacon Burst

Preparation Time : 10 minutes

Cooking Time: 90 minutes

Servings: 8

Ingredients

- ★ 30 slices bacon

- ★ 2 ½ cups cheddar cheese

- ★ 4-5 cups raw spinach

- ★ 1-2 tbsp Tones Southwest Chipotle Seasoning

- ★ 2 tsp Mrs. Dash Table

Seasoning Directions

1. Preheat your fryer to 375°F/190°C.

2. Weave the bacon into 15 vertical pieces & 12 horizontal pieces. Cut the extra 3 in half to fill in the rest, horizontally.

3. Season the bacon.

4. Add the cheese to the bacon.

5. Add the spinach and press down to compress.

6. Tightly roll up the woven bacon.

7. Line a baking sheet with kitchen foil and add plenty of salt to it.

8. Put the bacon on top of a cooling rack and put that on top of your baking sheet.

9. Bake for 60-70 minutes.

10. Let cool for 10-15 minutes before

11. Slice and enjoy!

Nutrition: calories 270, fat 15, fiber 3, carbs 5, protein 9

Grilled Ham & Cheese

Preparation Time: 10 minutes

Cooking Time: 30 minutes

Servings: 2

Ingredients

- ★ 3 low-carb buns

- ★ 4 slices medium-cut deli ham

- ★ 1 tbsp salted butter

- ★ 1 oz. flour

- ★ 3 slices cheddar cheese

- ★ 3 slices muenster

cheese Directions

Bread:

1. Preheat your fryer to 350°F/175°C.

2. Mix the flour, salt and baking powder in a bowl. Put to the side.

3. Add in the butter and coconut oil to a skillet.

4. Melt for 20 seconds and pour into another bowl.

5. In this bowl, mix in the dough.

6. Scramble two eggs. Add to the dough.

7. Add ½ tablespoon of coconut flour to thicken, and place evenly into a cupcake tray. Fill about ¾ inch.

8. Bake for 20 minutes until browned.

9. Allow to cool for 15 minutes and cut each in half for the buns.

Sandwich:

1. Fry the deli meat in a skillet on a high heat.

2. Put the ham and cheese between the buns.

3. Heat the butter on medium high.

4. When brown, turn to low and add the dough to pan.

5. Press down with a weight until you smell burning, then flip to crisp both sides.

6. Enjoy!

Nutrition:398

Calories; 21g

Fat; 4.7g

Carbs; 44.2g

Protein; 0

.5g Sugars

Prosciutto Spinach Salad

Preparation Time: 5 minutes

Cooking Time: 5 minutes

Servings: 2

Ingredients

- ★ 2 cups baby spinach
- ★ 1/3 lb prosciutto
- ★ 1 cantaloupe
- ★ 1 avocado
- ★ ¼ cup diced red onion handful of raw, unsalted

walnuts Directions

1. Put a cup of spinach on each plate.

2. Top with the diced prosciutto, cubes of balls of melon, slices of avocado, a handful of red onion and a few walnuts.

3. Add some freshly ground pepper, if you like.

4. Serve!

Nutrition:

Calories: 156 Fat: 8.01g Carbohydrate: 20.33g

Protein: 1.98g Sugar: 0.33g

Cholesterol: 0mg

Riced Cauliflower & Curry Chicken

Preparation Time: 10 minutes

Cooking Time: 30 minutes

Servings: 6

Ingredients

- ★ 2 lbs chicken (4 breasts)

- ★ 1 packet curry paste

- ★ 3 tbsp ghee (can substitute with butter)

- ★ ½ cup heavy cream

- ★ 1 head cauliflower (around 1

kg) Directions

1. In a large skillet, melt the ghee.

2. Add the curry paste and mix.

3. Once combined, add a cup of water and simmer for 5 minutes.

4. Add the chicken, cover the skillet and simmer for 18 minutes.

5. Cut a cauliflower head into florets and blend in a food processor to make the riced cauliflower.

6. When the chicken is cooked, uncover, add the cream and cook for an additional 7 minutes.

7. Serve!

Nutrition: Calories: 96 Fat: 8.8g

Carbohydrates: 5.12g Protein: 1.2g Sugar: 0.4g Cholesterol: 0mg

Mashed Garlic Turnips

Preparation Time: 5 minutes

Cooking Time: 10 minutes

Servings: 2

Ingredients

- ★ 3 cups diced turnip

- ★ 2 cloves garlic, minced

- ★ ¼ cup heavy cream

- ★ 3 tbsp melted butter

- ★ Salt and pepper to

season Directions

1. Boil the turnips until tender.

2. Drain and mash the turnips.

3. Add the cream, butter, salt, pepper and garlic. Combine well.

4. Serve!

Nutrition: Calories: 156 Fat: 8.01g

Carbohydrate: 20.33g

Protein: 1.98g

Sugar: 0.33g

Cholesterol: 0mg

Lasagna Spaghetti Squash

Preparation Time: 20 minutes

Cooking Time: 90 minutes

Servings: 6

Ingredients

- ★ 25 slices mozzarella cheese

- ★ 1 large jar (40 oz) Rao's Marinara sauce

- ★ 30 oz whole-milk ricotta cheese

- ★ 2 large spaghetti squash, cooked (44 oz)

- ★ 4 lbs ground beef

Directions 1. Preheat your fryer to 375°F/190°C.

2. Slice the spaghetti squash and place it face down inside a fryerproof dish. Fill with water until covered.

3. Bake for 45 minutes until skin is soft.

4. Sear the meat until browned.

5. In a large skillet, heat the browned meat and marinara sauce. Set aside when warm.

6. Scrape the flesh off the cooked squash to resemble strands of spaghetti.

7. Layer the lasagna in a large greased pan in alternating layers of spaghetti squash, meat sauce, mozzarella, ricotta. Repeat until all increased have been used.

8. Bake for 30 minutes and serve!

Nutrition: calories 270, fat 15, fiber 3, carbs 5, protein 9

Blue Cheese Chicken Wedges

Preparation Time: 10 minutes

Cooking Time: 45 minutes

Servings: 4

Ingredients

- ★ Blue cheese dressing

- ★ 2 tbsp crumbled blue cheese

- ★ 4 strips of bacon

- ★ 2 chicken breasts (boneless)

- ★ 3/4 cup of your favorite buffalo

sauce Directions

1. Boil a large pot of salted water.

2. Add in two chicken breasts to pot and cook for 28 minutes.

3. Turn off the heat and let the chicken rest for 10 minutes. Using a fork, pull the chicken apart into strips.

4. Cook and cool the bacon strips and put to the side.

5. On a medium heat, combine the chicken and buffalo sauce. Stir until hot.

6. Add the blue cheese and buffalo pulled chicken. Top with the cooked bacon crumble.

7. Serve and enjoy.

Nutrition: calories 270, fat 15, fiber 3, carbs 5, protein 9

'Oh so good' Salad

Preparation Time: 5 minutes

Cooking Time: 10 minutes

Servings: 2

Ingredients

- ★ 6 brussels sprouts

- ★ ½ tsp apple cider vinegar

- ★ 1 tsp olive/grapeseed oil

- ★ 1 grind of salt

- ★ 1 tbsp freshly grated

parmesan Directions

1. Slice the clean brussels sprouts in half.

2. Cut thin slices in the opposite direction.

3. Once sliced, cut the roots off and discard.

4. Toss together with the apple cider, oil and salt.

5. Sprinkle with the parmesan cheese, combine and enjoy!

Nutrition: calories 270, fat 15, fiber 3, carbs 5, protein 9

'I Love Bacon'

Preparation Time: 10 minutes

Cooking Time: 90 minutes

Servings: 4

Ingredients

- ★ 30 slices thick-cut bacon
- ★ 12 oz steak
- ★ 10 oz pork sausage
- ★ 4 oz cheddar cheese, shredded

Directions 1.Lay out 5 x 6 slices of bacon in a woven pattern and bake at 400°F/200°C for 20 minutes until crisp.

2.Combine the steak, bacon and sausage to form a meaty mixture.

3.Lay out the meat in a rectangle of similar size to the bacon strips. Season with salt/peppe.

4.Place the bacon weave on top of the meat mixture.

5.Place the cheese in the center of the bacon.

6.Roll the meat into a tight roll and refrigerate.

7.Make a 7 x 7 bacon weave and roll the bacon weave over the meat, diagonally.

8.Bake at 400°F/200°C for 60 minutes or 165°F/75°C internally.

9.Let rest for 5 minutes before serving.

Nutrition: Calories: 96 Fat: 8.8g Carbohydrates: 5.12g Protein: 1.2g Sugar: 0.4g Cholesterol: 0mg

Lemon Dill Trout

Preparation Time: 5 minutes

Cooking Time: 10 minutes

Servings: 1

Ingredients

- ★ 2 lb pan-dressed trout (or other small fish), fresh or frozen

- ★ 1 ½ tsp salt

- ★ ½ cup butter or margarine

- ★ 2 tbsp dill weed

- ★ 3 tbsp lemon

juice Directions

1. Cut the fish lengthwise and season the with pepper.

2. Preparation Timeare a skillet by melting the butter and dill weed.

3. Fry the fish on a high heat, flesh side down, for 2-3 minutes per side.

4. Remove the fish. Add the lemon juice to the butter and dill to create a sauce.

5. Serve the fish with the sauce.

Bell Peppers Stew

Preparation Time: 20 minutes

Servings: 4

Ingredients:

2 yellow bell peppers; cut into wedges

½ cup tomato sauce

2 red bell peppers; cut into wedges

2 green bell peppers; cut into wedges

1 tbsp. chili powder

¼ tsp. sweet paprika

2 tsp. cumin, ground

Salt and black pepper to taste.

Directions:

In a pan that fits your air fryer, mix all the ingredients, toss, introduce the pan in the machine and cook at 370°F for 15 minutes

Divide into bowls.

Nutrition: Calories: 190;

Fat: 4g;

Fiber: 2g;

Carbs: 4g;

Protein: 7g

Tomato and Avocado

Preparation Time: 8 minutes

Cooking Time: 15

Servings: 4

Ingredients:

- ★ ½ lb. cherry tomatoes; halved
- ★ 2 avocados, pitted; peeled and cubed
- ★ 1 ¼ cup lettuce; torn
- ★ 1/3 cup coconut cream
- ★ A pinch of salt and black pepper
- ★ Cooking

spray Directions:

Grease the air fryer with cooking spray, combine the tomatoes with avocados, salt, pepper and the cream and cook at 350°F for 5 minutes shaking once

In a salad bowl, mix the lettuce with the tomatoes and avocado mix, toss and serve.

Nutrition: Calories:

226; Fat: 12g;

Fiber: 2g;

Carbs: 4g;

Protein: 8g

Tomato Stew

Preparation Time: 20 minutes

Cooking Time: 15 minutes

Servings: 4

Ingredients:

- 25 oz. canned tomatoes; cubed

- 4 spring onions; chopped.

- 2 red bell peppers; cubed

- 1 tbsp. cilantro; chopped.

- 1 tsp. sweet paprika

- Salt and black pepper to

taste. Directions:

In a pan that fits your air fryer, mix all the ingredients, toss, introduce the pan in the fryer and cook at 360°F for 15 minutes

Divide into bowls and serve.

Nutrition:

Calories: 185;

Fat: 3g;

Fiber: 2g;

Carbs: 4g; Protein: 9g

Salmon and Kale Salad

Preparation Time: 13 minutes

Cooking Time: 10 minutes

Servings: 4

Ingredients:

* 4 salmon fillets; boneless

* 3 cups kale leaves; shredded

* 2 tbsp. olive oil

* 2 tsp. balsamic vinegar

* Salt and black pepper to

taste. Directions:

Put the fish in your air fryer's basket, season with salt and pepper, drizzle half of the oil over them, cook at 400°F for 4 minutes on each side, cool down and cut into medium cubes

Take a bowl and mix the kale with salt, pepper, vinegar, the rest of the oil and the salmon, toss gently and serve.

Nutrition:

Calories: 240;

Fat: 14g;

Fiber: 3g;

Carbs: 5g;

Protein: 10g

Pork Stew

Preparation Time: 35 minutes

Cooking Time: 25 minutes

Servings: 4

Ingredients:

- 2 lb. pork stew meat; cubed
- 1 eggplant; cubed
- ½ cup beef stock
- 2 zucchinis; cubed
- ½ tsp. smoked paprika
- Salt and black pepper to taste.
- A handful cilantro;

chopped. Directions:

In a pan that fits your air fryer, mix all the ingredients, toss, introduce in your air fryer and cook at 370°F for 30 minutes

Divide into bowls and serve right away.

Nutrition: Calories: 245; Fat: 12g;

Fiber: 2g;

Carbs: 5g;

Protein: 14g

Okra and Green Beans Stew

Preparation Time: 20 minutes

Cooking Time: 10 minutes

Servings: 4

Ingredients:

- ★ 1 lb. green beans; halved

- ★ 4 garlic cloves; minced

- ★ 1 cup okra

- ★ 3 tbsp. tomato sauce

- ★ 1 tbsp. thyme; chopped.

- ★ Salt and black pepper to

taste. Directions:

In a pan that fits your air fryer, mix all the ingredients, toss, introduce the pan in the air fryer and cook at 370°F for 15 minutes

Divide the stew into bowls and serve.

Nutrition:

Calories: 183;

Fat: 5g;

Fiber: 2g;

Carbs: 4g; Protein: 8g

Pork and Greens Bowls

Preparation Time: 25 minutes

Cooking Time: 10 minutes

Servings: 4

Ingredients:

- ½ lb. pork stew meat; cubed

- 2 cups mustard greens

- 2 green onions; chopped.

- ¼ cup tomato puree

- 1 yellow bell pepper; chopped.

- 1 tbsp. olive oil

- Salt and black pepper to

taste. Directions:

In a pan that fits your air fryer, mix all the ingredients, toss, introduce the pan in the air fryer and cook at 370°F for 20 minutes

Divide into bowls and serve.

Nutrition:

Calories: 265;

Fat: 12g;

Fiber: 3g; Carbs: 5g; Protein: 14g

Basil Chicken Bites

Preparation Time: 30 minutes

Cooking Time: 10 minutes

Servings: 4

Ingredients:

- ★ 1 ½ lb. chicken breasts, skinless; boneless and cubed
- ★ ½ cup chicken stock
- ★ ½ tsp. basil; dried
- ★ 2 tsp. smoked paprika
- ★ Salt and black pepper to

taste. Directions:

In a pan that fits the air fryer, combine all the ingredients, toss, introduce the pan in the fryer and cook at 390°F for 25 minutes

Divide between plates and serve for lunch with a side salad.

Nutrition:

Calories: 223;

Fat: 12g;

Fiber: 2g;

Carbs: 5g;

Protein: 13g

Mustard Chicken Thighs

Preparation Time: 35 minutes

Cooking Time: 15 minutes

Servings: 4

Ingredients:

- ★ 1 ½ lb. chicken thighs, bone-in

- ★ 2 tbsp. Dijon mustard

- ★ Cooking spray

- ★ A pinch of salt and black

pepper Directions:

Take a bowl and mix the chicken thighs with all the other ingredients and toss.

Put the chicken in your Air Fryer's basket and cook at 370°F for 30 minutes shaking halfway. Serve

Nutrition:

Calories: 253;

Fat: 17g;

Fiber: 3g;

Carbs: 6g;

Protein: 12g

Pork and Okra Stew

Preparation Time: 25 minutes

Cooking Time: 10 minutes

Servings: 4

Ingredients:

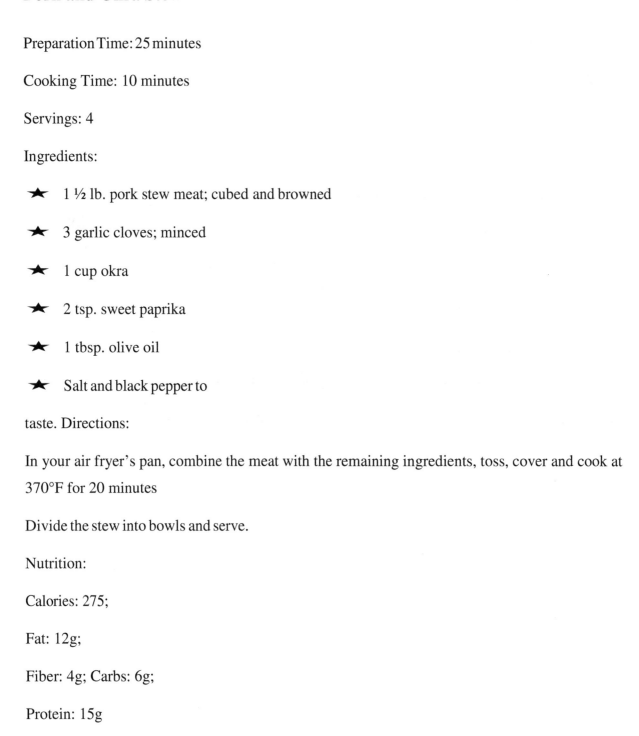

- 1 ½ lb. pork stew meat; cubed and browned

- 3 garlic cloves; minced

- 1 cup okra

- 2 tsp. sweet paprika

- 1 tbsp. olive oil

- Salt and black pepper to

taste. Directions:

In your air fryer's pan, combine the meat with the remaining ingredients, toss, cover and cook at 370°F for 20 minutes

Divide the stew into bowls and serve.

Nutrition:

Calories: 275;

Fat: 12g;

Fiber: 4g; Carbs: 6g;

Protein: 15g

Chicken Breast and Spring Onions

Preparation Time: 35 minutes

Cooking Time: 20 minutes

Servings: 4

Ingredients:

- ★ 4 spring onions; chopped.
- ★ 1 ½ cups parmesan cheese; grated
- ★ ½ cup tomato puree
- ★ 2 chicken breasts, skinless; boneless and cubed
- ★ 1 tsp. olive oil
- ★ Salt and black pepper to

taste. Directions:

Preheat your air fryer at 400°F, add half of the oil and the spring onions and fry them for 8 minutes, shaking the fryer halfway

Add the rest of the ingredients, toss, cook at 370°F for 22 minutes, shaking the fryer halfway as well.

Divide between plates and serve.

Nutrition:

Calories: 270;

Fat: 14g;

Fiber: 2g; Carbs: 6g; Protein: 12g

Spicy Chicken Enchilada Casserole

Preparation Time: 40 minutes

Cooking Time: 20 minutes

Servings: 2

Ingredients:

- ★ 1 lb. of chicken breasts, skinless and boneless
- ★ Salt and pepper to taste
- ★ ½ cup cilantro, fresh, minced
- ★ Olive oil spray
- ★ 2 cups cheddar cheese, shredded
- ★ Lime wedges (optional)
- ★ Sour cream (optional)
- ★ 1 (4-ounce) can of green chilies, chopped
- ★ 1 cup feta cheese, finely crumbled
- ★ 1 ½ cup enchilada sue

Directions:

Pat the chicken breasts dry and season with salt and pepper. Combine the chicken and enchilada sauce in a pan and simmer for 15-minutes over medium-low heat. Flip chicken over and cover and cook for an additional 15-minutes. Remove the chicken from pan and shred into bite-size pieces. Combine shredded chicken, feta cheese, enchilada sauce, chiles, and cilantro in a bowl. Add salt and pepper. Spray the air fryer baking dish with olive oil. Coat the entire bottom and sides. Evenly spread a cup of shredded cheese on the bottom of baking dish. Add the chicken mixture, then add another cup of cheese on top. Bake in your air fryer at 350°Fahrenheit for 10-minutes. Serve with optional lime wedges and sour cream.

Nutrition:

Calories: 338,

Total Fat: 12.3g,

Carbs: 8.3g,

Protein: 32.2g

Kale & Ground Beef Casserole

Preparation Time: 16 minutes

Cooking Time: 10 minutes

Servings: 4

Ingredients:

- ★ 4-ounces mozzarella, shredded
- ★ 2 cups marinara sauce
- ★ 10-ounces kale, fresh
- ★ 1 teaspoon oregano
- ★ 1 teaspoon onion powder
- ★ ½ teaspoon sea salt
- ★ 1 lb. lean ground beef

★ 2 tablespoons olive

Directions:

In a deep skillet, heat the olive oil for 2-minutes, add in the ground beef and cook for an additional 8-minutes or until meat is browned. Stir in salt, pepper, garlic powder, onion powder and oregano. In batches, stir the kale into beef mixture, cooking for another 2-minutes. Stir in the marinara sauce and cook for 2-minutes more. Mix in half the cheese into mixture. Transfer mixture into the air fryer baking dish. Sprinkle the remaining cheese on top. Broil in air fryer at 400°Fahrenheit for 2-minutes. Allow to rest for 5-minutes before serving.

Nutrition: Calories: 312, Total Fat: 13.2, Carbs: 9.2g, Protein: 43.2g

Cauliflower-Cottage Pie

Preparation Time: 40 minutes

Cooking Time: 20 minutes

Servings: 4

Ingredients:

★ Half a cup of bacon bits

★ 2 cups cauliflower rice

★ ¼ cup tomato puree

★ 1 tablespoon coconut oil

★ ½ white onion, chopped

★ 2lbs. lean ground beef

★ 1 tablespoon mixed spice blend

Directions:

In the frying pan add coconut oil and onions cook for 2-minutes. Add the ground beef into pan and cook for an additional 5-minutes or until meat is browned. Add spices and stir to combine. Add the tomato puree and mix well and cook for another 10-minutes. Transfer to air fryer baking dish. Top with cauliflower rice and bacon bits. Bake in air fryer at 350°Fahrenheit for 20-minutes. Serve warm.

Nutrition:

Calories: 367,

Total Fat: 13.4g,

Carbs: 11.2g,

Protein: 43.1g

DINNER RECIPES

Mustard Chicken Thighs

Preparation Time: 35 minutes

Cooking Time: 25 minutes

Servings: 4

Ingredients:

- ★ 1 ½ lb. chicken thighs, bone-in

- ★ 2 tbsp. Dijon mustard

- ★ Cooking spray

- ★ A pinch of salt and black

pepper Directions:

Take a bowl and mix the chicken thighs with all the other ingredients and toss.

Put the chicken in your Air Fryer's basket and cook at 370°F for 30 minutes shaking halfway. Serve

Nutrition::

Calories: 253;

Fat: 17g;

Fiber: 3g;

Carbs: 6g;

Protein: 12g

Tomato and Avocado

Preparation Time: 8 minutes

Cooking Time: 15 minutes

Servings: 4

Ingredients:

- ½ lb. cherry tomatoes; halved
- 2 avocados, pitted; peeled and cubed
- 1 ¼ cup lettuce; torn
- 1/3 cup coconut cream
- A pinch of salt and black pepper
- Cooking

spray Directions:

Grease the air fryer with cooking spray, combine the tomatoes with avocados, salt, pepper and the cream and cook at 350°F for 5 minutes shaking once

In a salad bowl, mix the lettuce with the tomatoes and avocado mix, toss and serve.

Nutrition:

Calories: 226;

Fat: 12g;

Fiber: 2g; Carbs: 4g;

Protein: 8g

Buttery Cod Bake

Preparation Time: 17 minutes

Cooking Time: 15 minutes

Servings: 4

Ingredients:

- ★ 2 cod fillets, boneless, skinless and cubed
- ★ ¼ cup tomato sauce
- ★ 8 cherry tomatoes; halved
- ★ 3 tbsp. butter; melted
- ★ 2 tbsp. parsley; chopped.
- ★ Salt and black pepper to

taste. Directions:

In a baking pan that fits the air fryer, combine all the ingredients, toss, put the pan in the machine and cook the mix at 390°F for 12 minutes

Divide the mix into bowls and serve for lunch.

Nutrition:

Calories: 232;

Fat: 8g;

Fiber: 2g;

Carbs: 5g; Protein: 11g

Broccoli Stew

Preparation Time: 20 minutes

Servings: 4

Ingredients:

- ★ 1 broccoli head, florets separated

- ★ ¼ cup celery; chopped.

- ★ ¾ cup tomato sauce

- ★ 3 spring onions; chopped.

- ★ 3 tbsp. chicken stock

- ★ Salt and black pepper to

taste. Directions:

In s pan that fits your air fryer, mix all the ingredients, toss, introduce the pan in your fryer and cook at 380°F for 15 minutes

Divide into bowls and serve for lunch.

Nutrition:

Calories: 183;

Fat: 4g;

Fiber: 2g;

Carbs: 4g;

Protein: 7g

Lemony Chicken Thighs

Preparation Time: 45 minutes

Cooking Time: 25 minutes

Servings: 6

Ingredients:

- ★ 3 lb. chicken thighs, bone-in

- ★ 1 tbsp. smoked paprika

- ★ ½ cup butter; melted

- ★ 1 tsp. lemon jice

Directions:

Take a bowl and mix the chicken thighs with the paprika, toss, put all the pieces in your air fryer's basket and cook them at 360°F for 25 minutes shaking the fryer from time to time and basting the meat with the butter.

Divide between plates and serve

Nutrition:

Calories: 261;

Fat: 16g;

Fiber: 3g;

Carbs: 5g;

Protein: 12g

Tomato Stew

Preparation Time: 20 minutes

Cooking Time: 35 minutes

Servings: 4

Ingredients:

- 25 oz. canned tomatoes; cubed

- 4 spring onions; chopped.

- 2 red bell peppers; cubed

- 1 tbsp. cilantro; chopped.

- 1 tsp. sweet paprika

- Salt and black pepper to

taste. Directions:

In a pan that fits your air fryer, mix all the ingredients, toss, introduce the pan in the fryer and cook at 360°F for 15 minutes

Divide into bowls and serve.

Nutrition:

Calories: 185;

Fat: 3g;

Fiber: 2g;

Carbs: 4g; Protein: 9g

Creamy Chicken

Preparation Time: 24 minutes

Cooking Time: 15 minutes

Servings: 4

Ingredients:

- ★ 4 chicken breasts, skinless; boneless and cubed

- ★ ¼ cup coconut cream

- ★ 1 ½ tsp. sweet paprika

- ★ 1 tsp. olive oil

- ★ Salt and black pepper to

taste. Directions:

Grease a pan that fits your air fryer with the oil, mix all the ingredients inside, introduce the pan in the fryer and cook at 370°F for 17 minutes

Divide between plates and serve.

Nutrition:

Calories: 250;

Fat: 12g;

Fiber: 2g;

Carbs: 5g;

Protein: 11g

Turkey and Mushroom Stew

Preparation Time: 30 minutes

Cooking Time: 25 minutes

Servings: 4

Ingredients:

- ★ ½ lb. brown mushrooms; sliced

- ★ 1 turkey breast, skinless, boneless; cubed and browned

- ★ ¼ cup tomato sauce

- ★ 1 tbsp. parsley; chopped.

- ★ Salt and black pepper to

taste. Directions:

In a pan that fits your air fryer, mix the turkey with the mushrooms, salt, pepper and tomato sauce, toss, introduce in the fryer and cook at 350°F for 25 minutes

Divide into bowls and serve for lunch with parsley sprinkled on top.

Nutrition:

Calories: 220;

Fat: 12g;

Fiber: 2g;

Carbs: 5g;

Protein: 12g

Basil Chicken Bites

Preparation Time: 30 minutes

Cooking Time: 15 minutes

Servings: 4

Ingredients:

- ★ 1 ½ lb. chicken breasts, skinless; boneless and cubed
- ★ ½ cup chicken stock
- ★ ½ tsp. basil; dried
- ★ 2 tsp. smoked paprika
- ★ Salt and black pepper to

taste. Directions:

In a pan that fits the air fryer, combine all the ingredients, toss, introduce the pan in the fryer and cook at 390°F for 25 minutes

Divide between plates and serve for lunch with a side salad.

Nutrition:

Calories: 223;

Fat: 12g;

Fiber: 2g;

Carbs: 5g;

Protein: 13g

Eggplant Bake

Preparation Time: 25 minutes

Cooking Time: 15 minutes

Servings: 4

Ingredients:

- ½ lb. cherry tomatoes; cubed

- ½ cup cilantro; chopped.

- 4 garlic cloves; minced

- 2 eggplants; cubed

- 1 hot chili pepper; chopped.

- 4 spring onions; chopped.

- 2 tsp. olive oil

- Salt and black pepper to

taste. Directions:

Grease a baking pan that fits the air fryer with the oil and mix all the ingredients in the pan.

Put the pan in the preheated air fryer and cook at 380°F for 20 minutes, divide into bowls and serve

Nutrition:

Calories: 232;

Fat: 12g; Fiber: 3g; Carbs: 5g;

Protein: 10g

Fennel and Tomato Stew

Preparation Time: 25 minutes

Cooking Time: 15 minutes

Servings: 4

Ingredients:

- ★ 2 fennel bulbs; shredded
- ★ ½ cup chicken stock
- ★ 1 red bell pepper; chopped.
- ★ 2 garlic cloves; minced
- ★ 2 cups tomatoes; cubed
- ★ 2 tbsp. tomato puree
- ★ 1 tsp. rosemary; dried
- ★ 1 tsp. sweet paprika
- ★ Salt and black pepper to

taste. Directions:

In a pan that fits your air fryer, mix all the ingredients, toss, introduce in the fryer and cook at 380°F for 15 minutes

Divide the stew into bowls.

Nutrition:

Calories: 184; Fat: 7g; Fiber: 2g; Carbs: 3g; Protein: 8g

Courgettes Casserole

Preparation Time: 25 minutes

Cooking Time: 15 minutes

Servings: 4

Ingredients:

- ★ 14 oz. cherry tomatoes; cubed
- ★ 2 spring onions; chopped.
- ★ 3 garlic cloves; minced
- ★ 2 courgettes; sliced
- ★ 2 celery sticks; sliced
- ★ 1 yellow bell pepper; chopped.
- ★ ½ cup mozzarella; shredded
- ★ 1 tbsp. thyme; dried
- ★ 1 tbsp. olive oil
- ★ 1 tsp. smoked

paprika Directions:

In a baking dish that fits your air fryer, mix all the ingredients except the cheese and toss.

Sprinkle the cheese on top, introduce the dish in your air fryer and cook at 380°F for 20 minutes. Divide between plates and serve for lunch

Nutrition: Calories: 254; Fat: 12g; Fiber: 2g; Carbs: 4g; Protein: 11g

Salmon and Kale Salad

Preparation Time: 13 minutes

Cooking Time: 15 minutes

Servings: 4

Ingredients:

- ★ 4 salmon fillets; boneless
- ★ 3 cups kale leaves; shredded
- ★ 2 tbsp. olive oil
- ★ 2 tsp. balsamic vinegar
- ★ Salt and black pepper to

taste. Directions:

Put the fish in your air fryer's basket, season with salt and pepper, drizzle half of the oil over them, cook at 400°F for 4 minutes on each side, cool down and cut into medium cubes

Take a bowl and mix the kale with salt, pepper, vinegar, the rest of the oil and the salmon, toss gently and serve.

Nutrition:

Calories: 240;

Fat: 14g;

Fiber: 3g;

Carbs: 5g;

Protein: 10g

Pork and Okra Stew

Preparation Time: 25 minutes

Cooking Time: 15 minutes

Servings: 4

Ingredients:

- ★ 1 ½ lb. pork stew meat; cubed and browned

- ★ 3 garlic cloves; minced

- ★ 1 cup okra

- ★ 2 tsp. sweet paprika

- ★ 1 tbsp. olive oil

- ★ Salt and black pepper to

taste. Directions:

In your air fryer's pan, combine the meat with the remaining ingredients, toss, cover and cook at 370°F for 20 minutes

Divide the stew into bowls and serve.

Nutrition:

Calories: 275;

Fat: 12g;

Fiber: 4g; Carbs: 6g;

Protein: 15g

Pork Stew

Preparation Time: 35 minutes

Cooking Time: 15 minutes

Servings: 4

Ingredients:

- 2 lb. pork stew meat; cubed

- 1 eggplant; cubed

- ½ cup beef stock

- 2 zucchinis; cubed

- ½ tsp. smoked paprika

- Salt and black pepper to taste.

- A handful cilantro;

chopped. Directions:

In a pan that fits your air fryer, mix all the ingredients, toss, introduce in your air fryer and cook at 370°F for 30 minutes

Divide into bowls and serve right away.

Nutrition:

Calories: 245;

Fat: 12g;

Fiber: 2g; Carbs: 5g; Protein: 14g

Cheese Eggplant Bowls

Preparation Time: 30 minutes

Cooking Time: 25 minutes

Servings: 4

Ingredients:

* ★ 1 cup mozzarella; shredded

* ★ 1 cup tomato puree

* ★ 2 cups eggplants; cubed

* ★ 1 tsp.

olive oil

Directions:

In a pan that fits the air fryer, combine all the ingredients except the mozzarella and toss.

Sprinkle the cheese on top, introduce the pan in the machine and cook at 390°F for 15 minutes. Divide between plates and serve

Nutrition:

Calories: 220;

Fat: 9g;

Fiber: 2g;

Carbs: 6g;

Protein: 9g

Turkey and Bok Choy

Preparation Time: 25 minutes

Cooking Time: 15 minutes

Servings: 4

Ingredients:

* 1 turkey breast, boneless, skinless and cubed

* 2 cups bok choy; torn and steamed

* 1 tbsp. balsamic vinegar

* 2 tsp. olive oil

* ½ tsp. sweet paprika

* Salt and black pepper to

taste. Directions:

Take a bowl and mix the turkey with the oil, paprika, salt and pepper, toss, transfer them to your Air Fryer's basket and cook at 350°F for 20 minutes

In a salad, mix the turkey with all the other ingredients, toss and serve.

Nutrition:

Calories: 250;

Fat: 13g;

Fiber: 3g;

Carbs: 6g; Protein: 14g

Chicken and Celery Stew

Preparation Time: 35 minutes

Cooking Time: 15 minutes

Servings: 6

Ingredients:

- ★ 1 lb. chicken breasts, skinless; boneless and cubed

- ★ 4 celery stalks; chopped.

- ★ ½ cup coconut cream

- ★ 2 red bell peppers; chopped.

- ★ 2 tsp. garlic; minced

- ★ 1 tbsp. butter, soft

- ★ Salt and black pepper to

taste. Directions:

Grease a baking dish that fits your air fryer with the butter, add all the ingredients in the pan and toss them.

Introduce the dish in the fryer, cook at 360°F for 30 minutes, divide into bowls and serve

Nutrition:

Calories: 246;

 Fat: 12g;

Fiber: 2g; Carbs: 6g; Protein: 12g

Mushroom Pork Chops

Preparation Time: 5-10 min.

Cooking Time: 15 min.

Servings: 4

Ingredients:

- ★ 2 tablespoon butter, melted

- ★ 1 pound pork chops, cut into small cubes

- ★ 8 ounce mushrooms, washed and halved

- ★ 1 teaspoon Worcestershire sauce or soy sauce

- ★ Black pepper and salt to taste

- ★ 1/2 teaspoon garlic

powder Directions:

1. In a mixing bowl, add the butter and seasoning. Combine the ingredients to mix well with each other. Add the mushroom and pork cubes; coat well.

2. Place Instant Pot Air Fryer Crisp over kitchen platform. Press Air Fry, set the temperature to 400°F and set the timer to 5 minutes to preheat. Press "Start" and allow it to preheat for 5 minutes.

3. In the inner pot, place the Air Fryer basket. In the basket, add the pork mixture.

4. Close the Crisp Lid and press the "Air Fry" setting. Set temperature to 400°F and set the timer to 14-18 minutes. Press "Start."

5. Halfway down, open the Crisp Lid, shake the basket and close the lid to continue cooking for the remaining time.

6. Open the Crisp Lid after cooking time is over. Cook for more time if not prepared for satisfaction. Season to taste and serve warm.

Nutrition: Calories: 456 Fat: 17.5g Saturated Fat: 2g Trans Fat: 0g

Carbohydrates: 23g Fiber: 4g Sodium: 196mg Protein: 34g

Meatball Meal Time

Preparation Time: 5-10 min.

Cooking Time: 15 min.

Servings: 6-8

Ingredients:

★ 2 tablespoon whole milk

★ 3 cloves garlic, minced

★ 1 tablespoon Dijon mustard

★ 1 shallot, minced

★ 2 tablespoon olive oil

★ 2/3 pound lean ground beef

★ 1 large egg, lightly beaten

★ 1/3 pound bulk turkey sausage

★ 1/4 cup flat-leaf parsley, chopped

★ 1 tablespoon thyme, chopped

★ 1 tablespoon rosemary, chopped

★ 1/2 teaspoon kosher

salt Directions:

1. Place Instant Pot Air Fryer Crisp over kitchen platform. Press "Sauté," select "Hi" setting and press "Start." In the inner pot, add the oil and allow it to heat.

2. Add the onions, garlic, and stir-cook until they become softened and translucent for 1-2 minutes.

3. In a mixing bowl, add the panko breadcrumbs and milk. Combine the ingredients to mix well with each other. Set aside for 5 minutes to soak.

4. Add the garlic and onion; combine well. Add the turkey sausage, beef, and the rest of the remaining ingredients—prepared small meatballs (1 ½ inch diameter) from the mixture.

5. Place Instant Pot Air Fryer Crisp over kitchen platform. Press Air Fry, set the temperature to 400°F and set the timer to 5 minutes to preheat. Press "Start" and allow it to preheat for 5 minutes.

6. In the inner pot, arrange trivet and place the Air Fryer basket. In the basket, add the meatballs.

7. Close the Crisp Lid and press the "Air Fry" setting. Set temperature to 400°F and set the timer to 10 minutes. Press "Start."

8. Halfway down, open the Crisp Lid, shake the basket and close the lid to continue cooking for the remaining time.

9. Open the Crisp Lid after cooking time is over. Serve warm.

Nutrition: Calories: 168 Fat: 7.5g

Saturated Fat: 1.5g Trans Fat: 0g Carbohydrates: 4g Fiber: 0g Sodium: 541mg Protein: 12g

Herbed Lamb Rack

Preparation Time: 5-10 min.

Cooking Time: 10 min.

Servings: 2

Ingredients:

- ★ 1 pound whole rack of lamb

- ★ 2 teaspoons garlic, minced

- ★ ½ teaspoon salt

- ★ 2 tablespoons rosemary, dried

- ★ 1 tablespoon thyme, dried

- ★ ½ teaspoon pepper

- ★ 4 tablespoons

olive oil Directions:

1. In a mixing bowl, add the olive oil and herbs. Combine the ingredients to mix well with each other. Coat the lamb with the herb mixture.

2. Place Instant Pot Air Fryer Crisp over kitchen platform. Press Air Fry, set the temperature to 400°F and set the timer to 5 minutes to preheat. Press "Start" and allow it to preheat for 5 minutes.

3. In the inner pot, place the Air Fryer basket. In the basket, add the lamb rack.

4. Close the Crisp Lid and press the "Air Fry" setting. Set temperature to 360°F and set the timer to 10 minutes. Press "Start."

5. Halfway down, open the Crisp Lid, shake the basket and close the lid to continue cooking for the remaining time.

6. Open the Crisp Lid after cooking time is over. Serve warm.

Nutrition: Calories: 542 Fat: 37g Saturated Fat: 9g

Trans Fat: 0.5g Carbohydrates: 3g Fiber: 0.5g Sodium: 693mg Protein: 45g

Baked Carrot Beef

Preparation Time: 5-10 min.

Cooking Time: 60 min.

Servings: 5-6

Ingredients:

- ★ 2 carrots, chopped

- ★ 2 sticks celery, chopped

- ★ 3 pounds beef

- ★ Olive oil to taste

- ★ 2 medium onions, sliced

- ★ Garlic cloves from 1 bunch

- ★ 1 bunch mixed fresh herbs (thyme, rosemary, bay, sage

etc.) Directions:

1. Grease a baking pan with some cooking spray. Add the vegetables, beef roast, olive oil, and herbs; combine well.

2. Place Instant Pot Air Fryer Crisp over kitchen platform. Press Air Fry, set the temperature to 400°F and set the timer to 5 minutes to preheat. Press "Start" and allow it to preheat for 5 minutes.

3. In the inner pot, place the Air Fryer basket. In the basket, add the pan.

4. Close the Crisp Lid and press the "Bake" setting. Set temperature to 380°F and set the timer to 60 minutes. Press "Start."

5. Open the Crisp Lid after cooking time is over. Serve warm.

Nutrition: Calories: 306 Fat: 21g Saturated Fat: 7g Trans Fat: 0g Carbohydrates: 10g Fiber: 3g Sodium: 324mg Protein: 32g

Garlic Roasted Pork Tenderloin

Preparation Time: 5-10 min.

Cooking Time: 18 min.

Servings: 5-6

Ingredients:

- ★ ¼ teaspoon ground black pepper

- ★ ¼ teaspoon garlic powder

- ★ ¼ teaspoon salt

- ★ 1 ½ pound pork tenderloin

- ★ 1 tablespoon olive oil

Directions:

1. In a mixing bowl, add the olive oil, black pepper, salt, and garlic powder. Combine the ingredients to mix well with each other. Rub the mixture evenly over the pork tenderloin.

2. Place Instant Pot Air Fryer Crisp over kitchen platform. Press Air Fry, set the temperature to 400°F and set the timer to 5 minutes to preheat. Press "Start" and allow it to preheat for 5 minutes.

3. In the inner pot, place the Air Fryer basket. In the basket, add the tenderloins.

4. Close the Crisp Lid and press the "Roast" setting. Set temperature to 400°F and set the timer to 25 minutes. Press "Start."

5. Halfway down, open the Crisp Lid, flip the tenderloin and close the lid to continue cooking for the remaining time.

6. Open the Crisp Lid after cooking time is over. Slice and serve warm.

Nutrition:

Calories: 203

Fat: 6g

Saturated Fat: 1.5g

Trans Fat: 0g

Carbohydrates: 2g

Fiber: 0g

Sodium: 173mg

Protein: 29g

Montreal Roast Beef

Preparation Time: 5-10 min.

Cooking Time: 15 min.

Servings: 6

Ingredients:

★   1 tablespoon olive oil

★   2 ½ pound beef

★   1 tablespoon Montreal steak

seasoning Directions:

1. Rub the olive oil over the beef roast. Rub with the seasoning.

2. Place Instant Pot Air Fryer Crisp over kitchen platform. Press Air Fry, set the temperature to 400°F and set the timer to 5 minutes to preheat. Press "Start" and allow it to preheat for 5 minutes.

3. In the inner pot, place the Air Fryer basket. In the basket, add the roast.

4. Close the Crisp Lid and press the "Roast" setting. Set temperature to 400°F and set the timer to 5 minutes. Press "Start."

5. Halfway down, open the Crisp Lid, flip the roast and close the lid to continue cooking for the remaining time.

6. Open the Crisp Lid after cooking time is over. Serve warm.

Nutrition:

Calories: 266 Fat: 12g Saturated Fat: 3g Trans Fat: 0.5g

Carbohydrates: 2.5g Fiber: 0g Sodium: 301mg Protein: 38g

Crisped Pork Chops

Preparation Time: 5-10 min.

Cooking Time: 15 min.

Servings: 4-6

Ingredients:

- ★ 2 beaten eggs

- ★ 4-6 thick boneless pork chops

- ★ 3 tablespoons grated parmesan cheese

- ★ 1 cup pork rind

- ★ 1 teaspoon smoked paprika

- ★ ¼ teaspoon pepper

- ★ ¼ teaspoon chili powder

- ★ ½ teaspoon onion powder

- ★ ½ teaspoon

salt Directions:

1. Season the pork chops with pepper and salt. Blend the rind in a blender or food processor to make rind crumbs.

2. In a mixing bowl, beat the eggs. Coat the chops with the eggs and then coat with the rind crumbs.

3. Place Instant Pot Air Fryer Crisp over kitchen platform. Press Air Fry, set the temperature to 400°F and set the timer to 5 minutes to preheat. Press "Start" and allow it to preheat for 5 minutes.

4. In the inner pot, place the Air Fryer basket. In the basket, add the chops.

5. Close the Crisp Lid and press the "Air Fry" setting. Set temperature to 400°F and set the timer to 5 minutes. Press "Start."

6. Halfway down, open the Crisp Lid, flip the chops and close the lid to continue cooking for the remaining time.

7. Open the Crisp Lid after cooking time is over. Serve warm.

Nutrition:

Calories: 391

Fat: 18g

Saturated Fat: 3.5g

Trans Fat: 0g

Carbohydrates: 17g

Fiber: 1.5g

Sodium: 547mg

Protein: 38g

POULTRY RECIPES

Turkey and Cream Cheese Breast Pillows

Preparation Time: 5 minutes.

Cooking time: 10 minutes.

Serving: 45

Ingredients:

- 1 cup of milk with 1 egg inside (put the egg in the cup and then fill with milk)

- 1/3 cup of water

- ¼ cup olive oil or oil

- 1 and ¾ teaspoon of salt

- 2 tbsp sugar

- 2 and ½ tbsp dried granular yeast

- 4 cups of flour

- 1 egg yolk to brush

- 2 jars of cream cheese

- 15 slices of turkey breast cut in 4

Direction:

1. *Mix all the dough ingredients with your hands until it is very smooth. After the ready dough, make small balls and place on a floured surface. Reserve*

2. *Open each dough ball with a roller trying to make it square. Cut squares of approximately 10 X 10 cm. Fill with a piece of turkey breast and 1 teaspoon of*

cream cheese coffee. Close the union of the masses joining the 4 points. Brush with the egg yolk and set aside.

3. Preheat the air fryer. Set the timer of 5 minutes and the temperature to 200C.

4. Place 6 units in the basket of the air fryer and bake for 4 or 5 minutes at 180C. Repeat until all the pillows have finished cooking.

Nutrition:

- Calories: 538

- Fat: 29.97g

- Carbohydrates: 22.69g

- Protein: 43.64g

- Sugar: 0.56g

- Cholesterol: 137mg

Chicken Wings

Preparation Time: 10 minutes.

Cooking time: 25 minutes.

Serve: 2

Ingredients:

- 10 chicken wings (about 700g)

- Oil in spay

- 1 tbsp soy sauce

- ½ tbsp cornstarch

- 2 tbsp honey

- 1 tbsp ground fresh chili paste

- 1 tbsp minced garlic

- ½ tsp chopped fresh ginger

- 1 tbsp lime sumo

- ½ tbsp salt

- 2 tbsp chives

Direction:

1. *Dry the chicken with a tea towel. Cover the chicken with the oil spray.*

2. *Place the chicken inside the hot air electric fryer, separating the wings towards the edge so that it is not on top of each other. Cook at 200ºC until the skin is crispy for about 25 min. Turn them around half the time.*

3. *Mix the soy sauce with cornstarch in a small pan. Add honey, chili paste, garlic, ginger, and lime sumo. Simmer until it boils and thickens. Place the chicken in a bowl, add the sauce and cover all the chicken. Sprinkle with chives.*

Nutrition:

- Calories: 81

- Fat: 5.4g

- Carbohydrates: 0g

- Protein: 7.46g

- Sugar: 0g

- Cholesterol: 23mg

Pickled Poultry

Preparation Time: 10 minutes.

Cooking time: 25 minutes.

Serving: 4

Ingredients:

- 600g of poultry, without bones or skin

- 3 white onions, peeled and cut into thin slices

- 5 garlic cloves, peeled and sliced

- 3 dl olive oil

- 1 dl apple cider vinegar

- ½ l white wine

- 2 bay leaves

- 5 g peppercorns

- Flour

- Pepper

- Salt

Direction:

1. Rub the bird in dice that we will pepper and flour

2. Put a pan with oil on the fire. When the oil is hot, fry the floured meat dice in it until golden brown. Take them out and reserve, placing them in a clay or oven dish. Strain the oil in which you have fried the meat

3. Preheat the oven to 170º C

4. Put the already cast oil in another pan over the fire. Sauté the garlic and onions in it. Add the white wine and let cook about 3 minutes. Remove the pan from the heat, add the vinegar to the oil and wine. Remove, rectify salt, and pour this mixture into the source where you had left the bird dice. Introduce the source in the oven, lower the temperature to 140ºC and bake for 1 and ½ hours. Remove the source from the oven and let it stand at room temperature

5. When the source is cold, put it in the fridge and let it rest a few hours before serving.

Nutrition:

- Calories: 232

- Fat: 15g

- Carbohydrates: 5.89g

- Protein: 18.2g

- Sugar: 1.72g

- Cholesterol: 141mg

Cordon Bleu Chicken Breast

Preparation Time: 10 minutes.

Cooking time: 40 minutes.

Serving: 6

Ingredients:

- 4 flattened chicken breasts

- 8 slices of ham

- 16 slices of Swiss cheese

- 2 tsp fresh thyme

- ¼ cup flour

- 1 cup of ground bread

- 2 tsp melted butter

- 2 eggs

- 1 clove garlic finely chopped

- pam cooking spray

Direction:

1. *Preheat the air fryer to 350 degrees Fahrenheit (180 °C), set timer to 5 minutes. Then, flatten chicken breasts.*

2. *Fill the chicken breasts with two slices of cheese, then 2 slices of ham and finally 2 slices of cheese and roll up. Use a stick if necessary, to save the shape.*

3. Mix the ground bread with the thyme, the garlic finely chopped, with the melted butter and with salt and pepper. Beat the eggs. Season the flour with salt and pepper.

4. Pass the chicken rolls first through the flour, then through the egg and finally through the breadcrumbs.

5. Bake until the breasts are cooked, about 20 minutes.

6. Alternatively, before putting the chicken breasts in the air fryer you can fry them in a little butter and then finish cooking in the air fryer for 13-15 minutes.

Nutrition:

- Calories: 387

- Fat: 20g

- Carbohydrates: 18g

- Protein: 33g

- Sugar: 0g

- Cholesterol: 42mg

Fried Chicken

Preparation Time: 15 minutes.

Cooking time: 25 minutes.

Serving: 4

Ingredients:

- 1kg of chicken chopped into small pieces

- Garlic powder

- Salt

- Ground pepper

- 1 little grated ginger

- 1 lemon

- Extra virgin olive oil

Direction:

1. *Put the chicken in a large bowl.*

2. *Add the lemon juice and pepper.*

3. *Add some grated ginger and mix well.*

4. *Leave 15 minutes in the refrigerator.*

5. *Add now a jet of extra virgin olive oil and mix.*

6. *Put the chicken in the air fryer, if it does not fit in a batch, it is put in two.*

7. *Select 180 degrees, 25 minutes.*

8. *Shake the baskets a few times so that the chicken rotates and is made on all sides.*

9. *If you want to pass the chicken for flour, before putting it in the basket and frying, you can do it.*

Nutrition:

- Calories: 4

- Fat: 3.3g

- Carbohydrates: 2.3g

- Protein: 2.5g

- Sugar: 0.1g

- Cholesterol: 8.8mg

Rolls Stuffed with Broccoli and Carrots with Chicken

Preparation Time: 15 minutes.

Cooking time: 25 minutes.

Serving: 4

Ingredients:

- 8 sheets of rice pasta

- 1 chicken breast

- 1 onion

- 1 carrot

- 150g broccolis

- 1 can of sweet corn

- Extra virgin olive oil

- Salt

- Ground pepper

- Soy sauce

- 1 bag of rice three delicacies

Direction:

1. Start with the vegetable that you have to cook previously, stop them, peel the carrot.

2. Cut the carrot and broccoli as small as you can. Add the broccolis and the carrot to a pot with boiling water and let cook a few minutes, they have to be tender, but not too much, that crunch a little.

3. Drain well and reserve.

4. Cut the onion into julienne.

5. Cut the breast into strips.

6. In the Wok, put some extra virgin olive oil.

7. Add to the wok when it is hot, the onion and the chicken breast.

8. Sauté well until the chicken is cooked.

9. Drain the corn and add to the wok along with the broccolis and the carrot.

10. Sauté so that the ingredients are mixed.

11. Add salt, ground pepper and a little soy sauce.

12. Mix well and let the filling cool.

13. Hydrate the rice pasta sheets.

14. Spread on the worktable and distribute the filling between the sheets of rice paste.

15. Assemble the rolls and paint with a little oil.

16. Put in the air fryer, those who enter do not pile up.

17. *Select 10 minutes 200 degrees.*

18. *When you have all the rolls made, the first ones will have cooled, because to solve it, you now place all the rolls already cooked inside the air fryer, now it does not matter that they are piled up.*

19. *Select 180 degrees, 5 minutes.*

20. *Make while the rice as indicated by the manufacturer in its bag.*

21. *Serve the rice with the rolls.*

Nutrition:

- Calories: 125

- Fat: 4.58g

- Carbohydrates: 16.83g

- Protein: 4.69g

- Sugar: 4.43g

- Cholesterol: 0mg

Preparation Time ime: 15 minutes.

Cooking time: 25 minutes.

Serving: 4

Ingredients:

- 8 wheat cakes

- 1 large roasted breast

- Grated cheese

- Sour sauce

- Guacamole

- Extra virgin olive oil

Direction:

1. *Extend the wheat cakes.*

2. *Stuffed with grated cheese and well-roasted chicken breast.*

3. *Form the flues and paint with extra virgin olive oil.*

4. *Place in batches in the air fryer and select 180 degrees, 5 minutes on each side or until you see the flutes golden.*

5. *Serve with sour sauce and guacamole.*

Nutrition:

- Calories: 325

- Fat: 7g

- Carbohydrates: 45g

- Protein: 13g

- Sugar: 7g

- Cholesterol: 0mg

Spicy Chicken Strips

Preparation Time: 5 minutes.
Cooking time: 12 minutes.
Serving: 5
Ingredients:

- 1 cup buttermilk

- 1½ tbsp hot pepper sauce

- 1 tsp salt

- ½ tsp black pepper, divided

- 1 pound boneless and skinless chicken breasts, cut into ¾ inch strips

- ¾ cup panko breadcrumbs

- ½ tsp salt

- ¼ tsp hot pepper, or to taste

- 1 tbsp olive oil

Direction:

1. *Put the buttermilk, hot sauce, salt and ¼ teaspoon of black pepper in shallow bowl. Add chicken strips and refrigerate for at least two hours. Put breadcrumbs, salt, and the remaining black pepper and hot pepper in another bowl; Add and stir the oil.*

2. *Remove the chicken strips from the marinade and discard the marinade. Put the strips, few at the same time, to the crumb mixture. Press the crumbs to the strips to achieve a uniform and firm cover.*

3. *Put half of the strips in single layer inside the basket. Cook at a temperature of 350°F for 12 minutes. Cook the rest when the first batch is cooked.*

Nutrition:

- Calories: 207

- Fat: 9g

- Carbohydrates: 5g

- Protein: 25g

- Sugar: 0g

- Cholesterol: 0mg

Chicken Breasts Covered With Parmesan Cheese

Preparation Time: 5 minutes.

Cooking time: 12 minutes.

Serving: 2

Ingredients:

- ¼ cup panko breadcrumbs

- ¼ cup grated Parmesan cheese

- ¼ tsp dried basil

- 1 tbsp olive oil

- 1 tbsp spicy mustard

- 1 tsp Worcestershire sauce

- 2 boneless and skinless chicken breasts

Direction:

1. *Put the breadcrumbs, cheese, and basil in a small, shallow bowl. Add and stir the oil until completely mixed. Combine mustard with Worcestershire sauce in small bowl. Put the mustard mixture on both sides of the breasts.*

2. *Put the chicken in the bowl with the crumb mixture and press the crumbs on both sides of the breasts to achieve a uniform and firm cover.*

3. *Put the chicken inside the basket. Cook at a temperature of 350°F for 21 to 25 minutes, turning halfway through cooking.*

Nutrition:

- Calories: 386

- Fat: 10g

- Carbohydrates: 5g

- Proteins: 29g

- Sugar: 0g

- Cholesterol: 73mg

Chicken In Wheat Cake With Aioli Sauce

Preparation Time: 10 minutes.
Cooking time: 35 minutes.
Serving: 4
Ingredients:

- 500g breaded chicken

- 4 wheat cakes

- Extra virgin olive oil

- 1 small lettuce

- Grated cheese

- Aioli sauce

Direction:

1. *Put the breaded chicken in the air fryer with a little extra virgin olive oil and fry at 180 degrees for 20 minutes.*

2. *Take out and reserve.*

3. *Chop the lettuce,*

4. *Put the wheat cakes on the worktable and distribute the chopped lettuce between them.*

5. *On the chopped lettuce spread the pieces of breaded chicken.*

6. *Cover with grated cheese and add some aioli sauce.*

7. *Close the wheat cakes and place on the baking sheet.*

8. *Take to the oven, 180 degrees, 15 minutes or until the cheese is melted.*

Nutrition:

- Calories: 91

- Fat: 9.83g

- Carbohydrates: 1.06g

- Protein: 0.19g

- Sugar: 0.07g

- Cholesterol: 0mg

Soy Chicken and Sesame, Breaded and Fried

Preparation Time: 10 minutes.

Cooking time: 50 minutes.

Serving: 4

Ingredients:

- 1 large chicken breast

- Egg

- Breadcrumbs

- Extra virgin olive oil

- Salt

- Ground pepper

- Soy sauce

- Sesame

Direction:

1. *Cut the breast into fillets and put in a bowl.*

2. *Season.*

3. *Add soy sauce and sesame. Flirt well and leave 30 minutes.*

4. *Beat the eggs and pass all the steaks through the beaten egg and the breadcrumbs.*

5. *With a silicone brush, permeate the fillets well on both sides.*

6. *Place on the grill of the air fryer and select 180 degrees, 20 minutes.*

7. *Make the fillets in batches so that they pile against each other.*

Nutrition:

- Calories: 373

- Fat: 18.30g

- Carbohydrates: 6.24g

- Proteins: 34.74g

- Sugars: 5.67g

- Cholesterol: 0 mg

Chicken with Provencal Herbs and Potatoes

Preparation Time: 10 minutes.
Cooking time: 55 minutes.
Serving: 2
Ingredients:

- 4 potatoes

- 2 chicken hindquarters

- Provencal herbs

- Salt

- Ground pepper

- Extra virgin olive oil

Direction:

1. *Peel the potatoes and cut into slices.*

2. *Pepper and put on the grid of the base air fryer.*

3. *Impregnate the chicken well with oil, salt and pepper and put some Provencal herbs.*

4. *Place the chicken on the potatoes.*

5. *Take the grill to the bucket of the air fryer and put inside.*

6. *Select 170 degrees 40 minutes.*

7. *Turn the chicken and leave 15 more minutes.*

Nutrition:

- Calories: 198.5

- Fat: 4.2g

- Carbohydrates: 17.6g

- Protein: 21.7g

- Sugar: 0.82g

Chicken Tears

Preparation Time: 15 minutes.

Cooking time: 25 minutes.

Serving: 4

Ingredients:

- 2 chicken breasts

- Flour

- Salt

- Ground pepper

- Extra virgin olive oil

- Lemon juice

- Garlic powder

Direction:

1. *Cut the chicken breasts into tears. Season and put some lemon juice and garlic powder. Let flirt well.*

2. *Go through flour and shake.*

3. *Place the tears in the basket of the air fryer and paint with extra virgin olive oil.*

4. *Select 180 degrees, 20 minutes.*

5. *Move from time to time so that the tears are made on all their faces.*

Nutrition:

- Calories: 197

- Fat: 8g

- Carbohydrates: 16g

- Protein: 14g

- Sugar: 0mg

- Cholesterol: 0mg

Breaded Chicken with Seed Chips

Preparation Time: 10 minutes.

Cooking time: 40 minutes.

Serving: 4

Ingredients:

- 12 chicken breast fillets

- Salt

- 2 eggs

- 1 small bag of seed chips

- Breadcrumbs

- Extra virgin olive oil

-

Direction:

1. *Put salt to chicken fillets.*

2. *Crush the seed chips and when we have them fine, bind with the breadcrumbs.*

3. *Beat the two eggs.*

4. *Pass the chicken breast fillets through the beaten egg and then through the seed chips that you have tied with the breadcrumbs.*

5. *When you have them all breaded, paint with a brush of extra virgin olive oil.*

6. *Place the fillets in the basket of the air fryer without being piled up.*

7. *Select 170 degrees, 20 minutes.*

8. *Take out and put another batch, repeat temperature and time. So, until you use up all the steaks.*

Nutrition:

- Calories: 242

- Fat: 13g

- Carbohydrates: 13.5g

- Protein: 18g

- Sugar: 0g

- Cholesterol: 42mg

Salted Biscuit Pie Turkey Chops

Preparation Time: 5 minutes.

Cooking time: 20 minutes.

Serving: 4

Ingredients:

- 8 large turkey chops

- 300 gr of crackers

- 2 eggs

- Extra virgin olive oil

- Salt

- Ground pepper

Direction:

1. *Put the turkey chops on the worktable, and salt and pepper.*

2. *Beat the eggs in a bowl.*

3. *Crush the cookies in the Thermomix with a few turbo strokes until they are made grit, or you can crush them with the blender.*

4. *Put the cookies in a bowl.*

5. *Pass the chops through the beaten egg and then passed them through the crushed cookies. Press well so that the empanada is perfect.*

6. *Paint the empanada with a silicone brush and extra virgin olive oil.*

7. *Put the chops in the basket of the air fryer, not all will enter. They will be done in batches.*

8. *Select 200 degrees, 15 minutes.*

9. *When you have all the chops made, serve.*

Nutrition:

- Calories: 126

- Fat: 6g

- Carbohydrates 0g

- Protein: 18g

- Sugar: 0g

Chicken Flutes with Sour Sauce and Guacamole

Preparation Time: 15 minutes.

Cooking time: 25 minutes.

Serving: 4

Ingredients:

- ☐ 8 wheat cakes

- ☐ 1 large roasted breast

- ☐ Grated cheese

- ☐ Sour sauce

- □ Guacamole

- □ Extra virgin olive oil

Direction:

1. Extend the wheat cakes.

2. Stuffed with grated cheese and well-roasted chicken breast.

3. Form the flues and paint with extra virgin olive oil.

4. Place in batches in the air fryer and select 180 degrees, 5 minutes on each side or until you see the flutes golden.

5. Serve with sour sauce and guacamole.

Nutrition:

□ Calories: 325

□ Fat: 7g

□ Carbohydrates: 45g

□ Protein: 13g

□ Sugar: 7g

□ Cholesterol: 0mg

Mustard Honey Chicken

Preparation Time: 5-10 min.

Cooking Time: 40 min.

Servings: 4

Ingredients:

- 4 chicken breasts

- ½ teaspoon paprika

- ½ teaspoon garlic powder

- 2 tablespoons sriracha

- 1 tablespoon honey

- 3 tablespoons rice vinegar

- 1 teaspoon Dijon mustard

- Black pepper (ground) and salt to taste

Directions:

1. Take a zip-lock bag, add all ingredients. Shake well and refrigerate for 2-3 hours to marinate.

2. Place Instant Pot over kitchen platform. Place Air Fryer Lid on top. Press Air Fry, set the temperature to 375°F and set the timer to 5 minutes to preheat. Press "Start" and allow it to preheat for 5 minutes.

3. Take Air Fryer Basket, grease it with some cooking spray. In the basket, add chicken.

4. Place the basket in the inner pot of Instant Pot, close Air Fryer Lid on top.

5. Press the "Air Fry" setting. Set temperature to 375°F and set the timer to 40 minutes. Press "Start." Flip chicken every 10 minutes.

6. Open Air Fryer Lid after cooking time is over. Serve warm.

Nutrition: Calories: 539 Fat: 26g Saturated Fat: 7.5g

Trans Fat: 0g Carbohydrates: 7g Fiber: 0.5g Sodium: 770mg Protein: 52g

Baked Tomato Chicken

Preparation Time: 5-10 min.

Cooking Time: 20 min.

Servings: 2

Ingredients:

- 3 tablespoons olive oil
- 1/2-pint grape tomatoes
- 6 pitted Greek olives, sliced
- 2 boneless skinless chicken breast halves
- 1/4 teaspoon salt
- 1/4 teaspoon pepper
- 2 tablespoons capers, drained

Directions:

1. Season chicken with ground black pepper and salt.

2. Place Instant Pot over kitchen platform. Place Air Fryer Lid on top. Press Air Fry, set the temperature to 375°F and set the timer to 5 minutes to preheat. Press "Start" and allow it to preheat for 5 minutes.

3. Take Air Fryer Basket, grease it with some cooking spray. In the basket, add the chicken. Add the remaining ingredients and stir.

4. Place the basket in the inner pot of Instant Pot, close Air Fryer Lid on top.

5. Press the "Bake" setting. Set temperature to 330°F and set the timer to 15 minutes. Press "Start."

6. Open Air Fryer Lid after cooking time is over. Serve warm.

Nutrition:

Calories: 331

Fat: 17g

Saturated Fat: 3g

Trans Fat: 0g

Carbohydrates: 7g

Fiber: 1g

Sodium: 547mg

Protein: 35g

Cranberry Turkey Meatballs

Preparation Time: 5-10 min.

Cooking Time: 20 min.

Servings: 4

Ingredients:

- 1 pound ground turkey

- 1 ½ tablespoons water

- 2 teaspoons cider vinegar

- 1/3 cup cranberry sauce

- ¼ pound ground bacon

- 1 1/2 tablespoons barbecue sauce

- 1 teaspoon salt and more to taste

Directions:

1. In a mixing bowl, add the bacon, turkey, and one teaspoon salt. Combine the ingredients to mix well with each other. Prepare 16 meatballs from the mixture.

2. Take a skillet or saucepan; add cranberry sauce, barbecue sauce, water, salt, and cider vinegar; heat it over the medium cooking flame for 3-4 minutes to thicken. Set aside.

3. Place Instant Pot over kitchen platform. Place Air Fryer Lid on top. Press Air Fry, set the temperature to 375°F and set the timer to 5 minutes to preheat. Press "Start" and allow it to preheat for 5 minutes.

4. Take Air Fryer Basket, grease it with some cooking spray. In the basket, add meatballs and thickened sauce.

5. Place the basket in the inner pot of Instant Pot, close Air Fryer Lid on top.

6. Press the "Air Fry" setting. Set temperature to 360°F and set the timer to 15 minutes. Press "Start." Stir the mixture every 5 minutes.

7. Open Air Fryer Lid after cooking time is over. Serve warm.

Nutrition:

Calories: 235

Fat: 11.5g

Saturated Fat: 4g

Trans Fat: 0g

Carbohydrates: 24.5g

Fiber: 1.5g

Sodium: 522mg

Protein: 27.5g

Baked Herbed Chicken

Preparation Time: 5-10 min.

Cooking Time: 12 min.

Servings: 4

Ingredients:

- 4 bone-in chicken thighs with skin

- 1/8 teaspoon dried oregano

- 1/8 teaspoon ground thyme

- 1/8 teaspoon garlic salt

- 1/8 teaspoon onion salt

- 1/8 teaspoon paprika

- 1/8 teaspoon ground black pepper

Directions:

1. In a mixing bowl, add the pepper, paprika, thyme, oregano, onion salt, and garlic salt. Combine the ingredients to mix well with each other. Add chicken and coat well.

2. Place Instant Pot over kitchen platform. Place Air Fryer Lid on top. Press Air Fry, set the temperature to 375°F and set the timer to 5 minutes to preheat. Press "Start" and allow it to preheat for 5 minutes.

3. Take Air Fryer Basket, grease it with some cooking spray. In the basket, add chicken skin side down.

4. Place the basket in the inner pot of Instant Pot, close Air Fryer Lid on top.

5. Press the "Bake" setting. Set temperature to 390°F and set the timer to 12 minutes. Press "Start." Flip the chicken halfway down.

6. Open Air Fryer Lid after cooking time is over. Serve warm.

Nutrition:

Calories: 184

Fat: 11g

Saturated Fat: 3.5g

Trans Fat: 0g

Carbohydrates: 2g

Fiber: 0g

Sodium: 427mg

Protein: 19g

Lemongrass Chicken

Preparation Time: 5-10 min.

Cooking Time: 40 min.

Servings: 6

Ingredients:

- 2 lemongrass stalks

- 1 teaspoon turmeric

- 3 shallots, chopped

- 3 cloves of garlic, minced

- Black pepper (ground) and salt to taste

- 3 pounds whole chicken

- 2 tablespoons fish sauce

Directions:

1. Take a zip-lock bag, add all ingredients. Shake well and refrigerate for 2-3 hours to marinate.

2. Place Instant Pot over kitchen platform. Place Air Fryer Lid on top. Press Air Fry, set the temperature to 375°F and set the timer to 5 minutes to preheat. Press "Start" and allow it to preheat for 5 minutes.

3. Take Air Fryer Basket, grease it with some cooking spray. In the basket, add chicken.

4. Place the basket in the inner pot of Instant Pot, close Air Fryer Lid on top.

5. Press the "Air Fry" setting. Set temperature to 390°F and set the timer to 40 minutes. Press "Start." Flip chicken every 10 minutes.

6. Open Air Fryer Lid after cooking time is over. Serve warm.

Nutrition:

Calories: 434

Fat: 15g

Saturated Fat: 1.5g

Trans Fat: 0g

Carbohydrates: 32g

Fiber: 6g

Sodium: 593mg

Protein: 38g

Baked Turkey Broccoli

Preparation Time: 5-10 min.

Cooking Time: 20 min.

Servings: 4

Ingredients:

- 1/2 (10 ounces) broccoli florets

- 1/2 cup shredded Cheddar cheese

- 1/2 cup cooked white rice

- 1 cup turkey meat, cooked and chopped

- 1/2 (7 ounces) package whole wheat crackers, crushed

- 1 1/2 teaspoons butter, melted

Directions:

1. In a bowl, mix well-melted butter and crushed crackers.

2. Place Instant Pot over kitchen platform. Place Air Fryer Lid on top. Press Air Fry, set the temperature to 375°F and set the timer to 5 minutes to preheat. Press "Start" and allow it to preheat for 5 minutes.

3. Take Air Fryer Basket, grease it with some cooking spray. In the basket, add turkey, broccoli, rice, and other ingredients. Combine well.

4. Add the cracker mixture on top.

5. Place the basket in the inner pot of Instant Pot, close Air Fryer Lid on top.

6. Press the "Bake" setting. Set temperature to 360°F and set the timer to 20 minutes. Press "Start." Cook until the top is light brown.

7. Open Air Fryer Lid after cooking time is over. Serve warm.

Nutrition:

Calories: 271

Fat: 11g

Saturated Fat: 3.5g

Trans Fat: 0g

Carbohydrates: 24g

Fiber: 2g

Sodium: 668mg

Protein: 17g

Soy Sauce Baked Chicken

Preparation Time: 5-10 min.

Cooking Time: 30 min.

Servings: 3-4

Ingredients:

- 1/4 cup white sugar

- 1/4 cup soy sauce

- 1 1/2 teaspoons cornstarch

- 1 1/2 teaspoons cold water

- 1/4 teaspoon ground ginger

- 1/8 teaspoon ground black pepper

- 4 skinless chicken thighs

- 2 tablespoons cider vinegar

- 1/2 clove garlic, minced

Directions:

1. Place Instant Pot over kitchen platform. Place Air Fryer Lid on top. Press Air Fry, set the temperature to 375°F and set the timer to 5 minutes to preheat. Press "Start" and allow it to preheat for 5 minutes.

2. Take Air Fryer Basket, grease it with some cooking spray. In the basket, add chicken and other ingredients. Combine well.

3. Place the basket in the inner pot of Instant Pot, close Air Fryer Lid on top.

4. Press the "Bake" setting. Set temperature to 380°F and set the timer to 30 minutes. Press "Start." Cover chicken with the sauce halfway down.

5. Open Air Fryer Lid after cooking time is over. Serve warm.

Nutrition:

Calories: 264

Fat: 9g

Saturated Fat: 1.5g

Trans Fat: 0g

Carbohydrates: 17g

Fiber: 3g

Sodium: 588mg

Protein: 24g

Drunken Orange Chicken

Preparation Time: 5-10 min.

Cooking Time: 40 min.

Servings: 6

Ingredients:

- 3 pounds chicken breasts

- 1/3 cup orange juice

- 2 tablespoons whole coriander seeds

- 2 tablespoons brown sugar

- 2 tablespoons honey

- 3 cloves of garlic, minced

- 1 shallot, minced

- ¼ cup tequila

- Black pepper (ground) and salt to taste

Directions:

1. Take a zip-lock bag, add all ingredients. Shake well and refrigerate for 2-3 hours to marinate.

2. Take a skillet or saucepan; add marinade liquid; heat it over the medium cooking flame for 5 minutes to thicken. Set aside.

3.Place Instant Pot over kitchen platform. Place Air Fryer Lid on top. Press Air Fry, set the temperature to 375°F and set the timer to 5 minutes to preheat. Press "Start" and allow it to preheat for 5 minutes.

4.Take Air Fryer Basket, grease it with some cooking spray. In the basket, add chicken.

5.Place the basket in the inner pot of Instant Pot, close Air Fryer Lid on top.

6.Press the "Air Fry" setting. Set temperature to 375°F and set the timer to 40 minutes. Press "Start." Flip chicken every 10 minutes.

7.Open Air Fryer Lid after cooking time is over. Serve warm with the thickened sauce on top.

Nutrition:

Calories: 441

Fat: 21g

Saturated Fat: 4g

Trans Fat: 0g

Carbohydrates: 14g

Fiber: 2g

Sodium: 951mg

Protein: 46.5g

Kale Tomato Chicken

Preparation Time: 5-10 min.

Cooking Time: 30 min.

Servings: 4

Ingredients:

- ½ cup cherry tomatoes halved

- ½ teaspoon Worcestershire sauce

- ¼ cup Greek yogurt

- ¼ cup Parmesan cheese, grated

- 3 tablespoons extra virgin olive oil

- 4 large chicken breasts, pounded

- 1 clove garlic, minced

- 1 large bunch kale, chopped

- Juice from 2 lemons

- Black pepper (ground) and salt to taste

Directions:

1. In a mixing bowl, add kale and tomatoes. Combine and refrigerate for 2 hours. In another bowl, add other ingredients and combine well.

2. Place Instant Pot over kitchen platform. Place Air Fryer Lid on top. Press Air Fry, set the temperature to 375°F and set the timer to 5 minutes to preheat. Press "Start" and allow it to preheat for 5 minutes.

3. Take Air Fryer Basket, grease it with some cooking spray. In the basket, add chicken mixture.

4. Place the basket in the inner pot of Instant Pot, close Air Fryer Lid on top.

5. Press the "Air Fry" setting. Set temperature to 390°F and set the timer to 30 minutes. Press "Start."

6. Open Air Fryer Lid after cooking time is over. Slice the chicken, add and combine kale mixture. Serve warm.

Nutrition:

Calories: 469

Fat: 15g

Saturated Fat: 6.5g

Trans Fat: 0g

Carbohydrates: 7g

Fiber: 1g

Sodium: 748mg

Protein: 51g

Smoked BBQ Chicken

Preparation Time: 5-10 min.

Cooking Time: 30 min.

Servings: 8

Ingredients:

4 pounds chicken wings

- ½ cup barbecue sauce

- 1 tablespoon liquid smoke seasoning

- 3 tablespoons paprika

- 1 tablespoon garlic powder

- 1 teaspoon chipotle chili powder

- 4 teaspoons salt

- 1 tablespoon chili powder

- 1 teaspoon mustard powder

Directions:

1. Take a zip-lock bag, add all ingredients. Shake well and refrigerate for 2-3 hours to marinate.

2. Place Instant Pot over kitchen platform. Place Air Fryer Lid on top. Press Air Fry, set the temperature to 375°F and set the timer to 5 minutes to preheat. Press "Start" and allow it to preheat for 5 minutes.

3. Take Air Fryer Basket, grease it with some cooking spray. In the basket, add chicken mixture (reserve marinade).

4. Place the basket in the inner pot of Instant Pot, close Air Fryer Lid on top.

5. Take a skillet or saucepan; add marinade; heat it over the medium cooking flame for 5 minutes to thicken. Set aside.

6. Press the "Air Fry" setting. Set temperature to 390°F and set the timer to 30 minutes. Press "Start." Flip chicken every 10 minutes.

7. Open Air Fryer Lid after cooking time is over. Serve warm with the thickened marinade on top.

Nutrition:

Calories: 388

Fat: 9g

Saturated Fat: 1g

Trans Fat: 0g

Carbohydrates: 12g

Fiber: 0.5g

Sodium: 820mg

Protein: 48g

Oregano Whole Chicken

Preparation Time: 5-10 min.

Cooking Time: 18 min.

Servings: 6-8

Ingredients:

- 3 pound whole chicken, cut into 8 pieces
- 2 teaspoons onion powder
- 2 teaspoons garlic powder
- 1 teaspoon oregano dried
- 1 tablespoon thyme, dried
- ½ teaspoon ground black pepper
- ½ teaspoon kosher salt
- 1 teaspoon paprika, smoked
- ¼ teaspoon cayenne

Directions:

1. Rub the black pepper and salt evenly over the chicken. In a mixing bowl, combine cayenne, paprika, garlic powder, onion powder, oregano, and thyme. Add the chicken and coat well.

2. Grease Air Fryer Basket with some cooking spray. Add the chicken pieces.

3. Place Instant Pot Air Fryer Crisp over kitchen platform. Press Air Fry, set the temperature to 400°F and set the timer to 5 minutes to preheat. Press "Start" and allow it to preheat for 5 minutes.

4. In the inner pot, place the Air Fryer basket.

5. Close the Crisp Lid and press the "Air Fry" setting. Set temperature to 350°F and set the timer to 18 minutes. Press "Start."

6. Halfway down, open the Crisp Lid, shake the basket and close the lid to continue cooking for the remaining time.

7. Open the Crisp Lid after cooking time is over. Serve warm with your choice of dip.

Nutrition:

Calories: 208

Fat: 5g

Saturated Fat: 1g

Trans Fat: 0g

Carbohydrates: 3

Fiber: 0.5g

Sodium: 233mg

Protein: 34g

Mustard Turkey

Preparation Time: 5-10 min.

Cooking Time: 35 min.

Servings: 4

Ingredients:

- 2 pound turkey breast

- 1 teaspoon coarsely chopped sage

- 1 teaspoon chopped thyme

- 1 teaspoon finely chopped rosemary

- 1 tablespoon butter

- ¾ teaspoon ground black pepper

- ¼ cup maple syrup

- 2 tablespoons Dijon mustard

- ½ teaspoon kosher salt

Directions:

1. Season the turkey with black pepper and salt. Evenly rub the thyme, rosemary, and sage over the turkey.

2. In a mixing bowl, combine the melted butter, Dijon mustard, maple syrup.

3. Grease Air Fryer Basket with some cooking spray. Add the seasoned turkey.

4. Place Instant Pot Air Fryer Crisp over kitchen platform. Press Air Fry, set the temperature to 400°F and set the timer to 5 minutes to preheat. Press "Start" and allow it to preheat for 5 minutes.

5. In the inner pot, place the Air Fryer basket.

6. Close the Crisp Lid and press the "Air Fry" setting. Set temperature to 390°F and set the timer to 35 minutes. Press "Start."

7. Halfway down, open the Crisp Lid, shake the basket and close the lid to continue cooking for the remaining time.

8. Open the Crisp Lid after cooking time is over. Spread the maple syrup over the turkey and Air Fry for 2-3 more minutes. Serve warm.

Nutrition:

Calories: 426

Fat: 18g

Saturated Fat: 5g

Trans Fat: 0g

Carbohydrates: 14g

Fiber: 1.5g

Sodium: 523mg

Protein: 48g

Lemon Chicken Potatoes

Preparation Time: 5-10 min.

Cooking Time: 20 min.

Servings: 5-6

Ingredients:

½ cup chicken broth

12 chicken thighs, bone-in

1 ½ pound yellow potatoes, quartered

⅓ cup olive oil

⅓ cup lemon juice

1 teaspoon lemon zest

1 teaspoon dried parsley

1 teaspoon black pepper

1 tablespoon garlic, minced

2 teaspoons dried oregano

2 teaspoons kosher salt

Lemon wedges to serve

Directions:

1. In a mixing bowl, whisk the lemon juice, olive oil, garlic, parsley, oregano, pepper, lemon zest, and salt.

2. Place Instant Pot Air Fryer Crisp over kitchen platform. In the inner pot, add the broth and chicken. Arrange the potatoes on top and pour the lemon mixture.

3. Close the Pressure Lid and press the "Pressure" setting. Set the "Hi" pressure level and set the timer to 15 minutes. Press "Start."

4. Instant Pot will start building pressure. Quick-release pressure after cooking time is over (just press the button on the lid), and open the lid. Add the chicken mixture to a serving plate along with the lemon sauce.

5. Add back the chicken to the pot. Close the Crisp Lid and press the "Air Fry" setting. Set temperature to 400°F and set the timer to 4 minutes. Press "Start."

6. Halfway down, open the Crisp Lid, shake the basket and close the lid to continue cooking for the remaining time.

7. Open the Crisp Lid after cooking time is over. Add the chicken to the potato mixture and serve warm.

Nutrition:

Calories: 612

Fat: 38.5g

Saturated Fat: 12g

Trans Fat: 0g

Carbohydrates: 23g

Fiber: 6g

Sodium: 983mg

Protein: 43g

Classic Honey Mustard Chicken

Preparation Time: 5-10 min.

Cooking Time: 20 min.

Servings: 5-6

Ingredients:

- 3 tablespoons honey

- 2 tablespoons Dijon mustard

- 6 (6-ounces each) boneless, skinless chicken breasts

- 2 tablespoons rosemary, minced

- ¼ teaspoon ground black pepper

- ¾ teaspoon salt

Directions:

1. In a mixing bowl, combine the honey, Dijon mustard, black pepper, rosemary, and salt. Rub the chicken breasts with the mixture.

2. Grease Air Fryer Basket with some cooking spray. Arrange the chicken breasts.

3. Place Instant Pot Air Fryer Crisp over kitchen platform. Press Air Fry, set the temperature to 400°F and set the timer to 5 minutes to preheat. Press "Start" and allow it to preheat for 5 minutes.

4. In the inner pot, place the Air Fryer basket.

5. Close the Crisp Lid and press the "Air Fry" setting. Set temperature to 350°F and set the timer to 20-22 minutes. Press "Start."

6. Halfway down, open the Crisp Lid, shake the basket and close the lid to continue cooking for the remaining time.

7. Open the Crisp Lid after cooking time is over. Serve warm with veggies or cooked rice.

Nutrition:

Calories:

Fat: g

Saturated Fat: g

Trans Fat: 0g

Carbohydrates: g

Fiber: g

Sodium: mg

Protein: g

Broiled Italian Chicken

Preparation Time: 5-10 min.

Cooking Time: 20 min.

Servings: 4

Ingredients:

¾ cup shredded parmesan

1 cup panko breadcrumbs

4 chicken thighs with bone and skin

2 eggs, large

1 teaspoon Italian seasoning

½ teaspoon ground black pepper

1 teaspoon garlic powder

½ teaspoon kosher salt

Directions:

1. Rub black pepper and salt over the chicken. In a mixing bowl, combine the panko breadcrumbs, Italian seasoning, garlic powder, and parmesan.

2. Beat the eggs in another bowl. Coat the chicken first with the egg, then with the crumb mixture.

3. Place Instant Pot Air Fryer Crisp over kitchen platform. Press Air Fry, set the temperature to 400°F and set the timer to 5 minutes to preheat. Press "Start" and allow it to preheat for 5 minutes.

4. In the inner pot, place the Air Fryer basket. In the basket, add the chicken.

5. Close the Crisp Lid and press the "Broil" setting. Set temperature to 400°F and set the timer to 20 minutes. Press "Start." No need to flip in between.

6. Open the Crisp Lid after cooking time is over. Serve warm.

Nutrition:

Calories: 577

Fat: 32g

Saturated Fat: 9.5g

Trans Fat: 0g

Carbohydrates: 14g

Fiber: 1.5g

Sodium: 624mg

Protein: 42g

Asian Style Chicken Meal

Preparation Time: 5-10 min.

Cooking Time: 30 min.

Servings: 2-3

Ingredients:

- ¼ cup honey

- ½ cup rice vinegar

- 1 pound chicken wings

- 1 teaspoon sea salt

- 2 cloves garlic, minced

- 1 teaspoon ginger, grated

- 1 small orange, zest, and juice

- 2 teaspoons red chili pepper paste

Directions:

1. Place Instant Pot Air Fryer Crisp over kitchen platform. In the inner pot, add 2 cups water and arrange trivet and place the chicken wings over.

2. Close the Pressure Lid and press the "Pressure" setting. Set the "Hi" pressure level and set the timer to 2 minutes. Press "Start."

3. Instant Pot will start building pressure. Quick-release pressure after cooking time is over (just press the button on the lid), and open the lid. Take out the wings and empty water.

4. In a mixing bowl, combine the orange zest, orange juice, rice vinegar, honey, red pepper paste, ginger, garlic, and salt.

5. Add the sauce in the pot and place trivet; place the chicken over the trivet.

6. Close the Crisp Lid and press the "Air Fry" setting. Set temperature to 390°F and set the timer to 30 minutes. Press "Start."

7. Halfway down, open the Crisp Lid, shake the basket and close the lid to continue cooking for the remaining time.

8. Open the Crisp Lid after cooking time is over. Serve the chicken with the honey sauce.

Nutrition:

Calories: 448

Fat: 17g

Saturated Fat: 6g

Trans Fat: 0.5g

Carbohydrates: 41g

Fiber: 2g

Sodium: 1087mg

Protein: 24g

Chicken Air Fried with Pepper Sauce

Preparation Time: 5-10 min.

Cooking Time: 30 min.

Servings: 7-8

Ingredients:

- 1 tablespoon Worcestershire sauce

- 1 teaspoon salt

- 1-2 tablespoon brown sugar

- ½ cup cayenne pepper sauce

- 4 pounds chicken wings

- ½ cup butter

- Directions:

1. In a mixing bowl, add the salt, brown sugar, Worcestershire sauce, butter, and hot sauce. Combine the ingredients to mix well with each other.

2. Grease Air Fryer Basket with some cooking spray. Add the chicken wings.

3. Place Instant Pot Air Fryer Crisp over kitchen platform. Press Air Fry, set the temperature to 400°F and set the timer to 5 minutes to preheat. Press "Start" and allow it to preheat for 5 minutes.

4. In the inner pot, place the Air Fryer basket.

5. Close the Crisp Lid and press the "Air Fry" setting. Set temperature to 380°F and set the timer to 25 minutes. Press "Start."

6. Halfway down, open the Crisp Lid, shake the basket and close the lid to continue cooking for the remaining time.

7. Open the Crisp Lid after cooking time is over. Add it with the bowl sauce and combine; serve warm.

Nutrition:

Calories: 387

Fat: 15g

Saturated Fat: 5g

Trans Fat: 0g

Carbohydrates: 12g

Fiber: 0.5g

Sodium: 586mg

PORK RECIPES

Maple Ginger Pork Tenderloin

Preparation Time: 10 minutes + 2 hours marinating

Cooking Time: 30 minutes;

Serving: 4

Ingredients:

- ★ 1 ½ tbsp fresh grated ginger

- ★ 7 tbsp maple syrup

- ★ 2 freshly squeezed lemon juice

- ★ 2 tsp pressed garlic

- ★ 2 ½ tbsp soy sauce

- ★ Salt and black pepper to taste

- ★ A pinch cayenne pepper

- ★ 1 lb. pork tenderloin, excess fat trimmed

- ★ Olive oil for brushing

- ★ 2 tbsp chopped fresh chives for

garnishingDirections:

1. In a medium bowl, mix all the ingredients up to the pork and pour into a large zipper bag. Add the pork, seal the bag, and rub the marinade well onto the meat. Allow marinating in the refrigerator for 2 hours.

2.Once done marinating, heat 1 tbsp of the olive oil in a large skillet, remove the pork from marinade, and sear in the oil on both sides until golden brown, 3 to 4 minutes per side.

3.Meanwhile, insert the dripping pan onto the bottom part of the oven and preheat at Roast mode at 400 F for 2 to 3 minutes.

4.When the pork is ready, transfer to the cooking tray and brush all around with a little more olive oil. Slide the cooking tray onto the middle rack of the oven and close.

5.Set the timer to 10 to 15 minutes depending on your desired doneness, and press Start.

6.After the cooking time ends, slide out the tray, baste the meat with the leftover marinade, turn the meat over, and cook further for 1 to 2 minutes in the same setting or until golden brown.

7.Remove the meat from the oven and cover with foil and allow resting for 5 minutes before slicing.

8.Garnish with the chives and serve warm.

Nutrition:

Calories 301,

Total Fat 5.94g,

Total Carbs 30.65g,

Fiber 0.7g,

Protein 31.11g,

Sugar 24.91g,

Sodium 222mg

Honey Glazed Pork Shoulder

Preparation Time: 12 minutes + 2 hour marinating;

Cooking Time: 67 minutes;

Serving: 4

Ingredients:

- ★ 1 tsp fennel seeds, crushed
- ★ Salt to taste
- ★ ¼ cup brown sugar
- ★ 1 tsp whole black peppercorns, crushed
- ★ 6 lbs. skinless bone-in pork shoulder
- ★ ¼ cup + 1 tbsp apple cider vinegar
- ★ ¼ cup honey
- ★ ½ tsp black

pepper Directions:

1. In a small bowl, mix the fennel seeds, salt, brown sugar, and peppercorns. Rub the spice mix on both sides of the pork, cover with plastic wrap, and set aside to marinate for at least 2 hours.

2. When done marinating, preheat the oven at Bake mode at 400 F for 2 to 3 minutes.

3. Replace the pork cover with foil (meanwhile shaking off some of the rub before wrapping), place on the cooking tray and slide the tray onto the middle rack of the air fryer oven. Also, fill the dripping pan with water, carefully place on the bottom of the oven and close.

4. Set the timer for 1 hour, and cook until the timer reads to the end. If the meat isn't tender, cook further for 30 to 45 minutes.

5. Meanwhile, in a small bowl, whisk the apple cider vinegar, honey, and black pepper to make the glaze. Set aside.

6. When the meat is ready, remove the cooking tray, unwrap the pork, brush the top with the glaze, and return the meat to the oven.

7. Cook further in the same mode but for 12 minutes or until golden brown.

8. Transfer the meat to a clean, flat surface, allow sitting for 10 minutes before slicing.

9. Serve warm.

Nutrition:

Calories 991,

Total Fat 23.28g,

Total Carbs 33.27g,

 Fiber 0.4g,

Protein 153.62g,

Sugar 32.31g,

Sodium 374mg

Memphis Style Pork Ribs

Preparation Time: 10 minutes;

Cooking Time: 38 minutes;

Serving: 4

Ingredients:

- ★ 1 tsp garlic powder

- ★ 1 tsp onion powder

- ★ 1 tbsp salt

- ★ ½ tsp black pepper

- ★ 1 tsp beef seasoning

- ★ ½ tsp mustard powder

- ★ 1 tbsp dark brown sugar

- ★ 1 tbsp sweet paprika

- ★ 2 ¼ lbs. pork spareribs,

individually cut Directions:

1. Insert the dripping pan onto the bottom part of the oven and preheat at Air Fry mode at 350 F for 2 to 3 minutes.

2. In a small bowl, mix all the ingredients up to the spare ribs and them and rub the spice mixture on all sides of each rib.

3. Arrange the 4 to 6 ribs on the cooking tray, slide the tray onto the middle rack of the oven, and close the oven.

4. Set the timer for 35 minutes, and press Start. Cook until the ribs are golden brown and tender within while flipping every halfway.

5. Transfer to a plate when ready and allow cooling for 2 to 3 minutes before serving.

Nutrition: Calories 618, Total Fat 35.7g, Total Carbs 2.23g, Fiber 0.9g, Protein 67.75g, Sugar 0.24g, Sodium 1899mg

Thyme Roasted Pork Chops

Preparation Time: 10 minutes;

Cooking Time: 25 minutes;

Serving: 4

Ingredients:

- ★ 4 pork chops bone-in, loin, about 3/4-inch thickness

- ★ 1 tbsp olive oil

- ★ ¼ tsp garlic powder

- ★ ¼ tsp dried thyme

- ★ Salt and black pepper to

taste Directions:

1. Insert the dripping pan onto the bottom part of the oven and preheat at Roast mode at 400 F for 2 to 3 minutes.

2.Brush the meat on both sides with olive oil and season with the garlic powder, thyme, salt, and black pepper. Place two chops on the cooking tray, slide the tray onto the middle rack of oven and close.

3.Set the timer to 20 or 25 minutes depending on your desired doneness and press Start. Cook until the timer ends or until the meat is golden brown and tender within while flipping halfway.

4.Transfer to serving plates and cook the other two chops in the same manner.

5.Serve the chops immediately with buttered vegetables.

Nutrition:

Calories 363,

Total Fat 20.76g,

Total Carbs 1.22g,

Fiber 0.2g,

Protein 40.47g,

Sugar 0.58g,

Sodium 87mg

Bake Barbecued Pork Chops

Preparation Time: 10 minutes;

Cooking Time: 52 minutes;

Serving: 4

Ingredients:

- ★ 4 bone-in pork chops, thick cut
- ★ Salt and black pepper to taste
- ★ ½ tsp garlic powder
- ★ ¼ tsp cayenne pepper
- ★ ¼ cup brown sugar
- ★ 2 tbsp honey
- ★ 1 cup ketchup
- ★ ½ cup hot sauce
- ★ 1 tsp apple cider vinegar
- ★ ½ tsp paprika
- ★ 1 tbsp Worcestershire sauce
- ★ 1 tbsp yellow mustard
- ★ ¼ tsp celery salt

Directions:

1. Preheat the oven at Bake mode at 350 F for 2 to 3 minutes and lightly grease an 8-inch baking dish (safe for the air fryer) with olive oil. Set aside.

2. Season the pork chops with salt, black pepper, and lay in the baking dish.

3. In a small bowl, mix the remaining ingredients and pour the mixture all over the meat while lifting the meat a little to have some of the spice mix go under the chops. Cover the dish with foil.

4. Slide the cooking tray upside down on the middle rack of the oven, place the baking dish on top and close the air fryer.

5. Set the timer for 45 or 50 minutes, and press Start. Cook until the timer reads to the end while opening the dish and turning the meat.

6. Once the timer ends, take off the foil, set the air fryer in Broil mode and press Start to brown the top of the pork.

7. When ready, remove the dish from the oven, allow sitting for 2 minutes and serve afterwards.

Nutrition:

Calories 489,

Total Fat 17.75g,

Total Carbs 41.74g,

Fiber 0.8g,

Protein 41.52g,

Sugar 0.02g,

Sodium 1482mg

Pork Chops with Chicory Treviso

Preparation Time: 10-20;

Cooking time: 0-15;

Serving: 2

Ingredients:

★ ☐ 4 pork chops

★ ☐ 40g butter

★ ☐ Flour to taste

★ ☐ 1 chicory stalk

★ ☐ Salt to taste

Direction:

1. Cut the chicory into small pieces. Place the butter and chicory in pieces on the basket of the air fryer previously preheated at 1800C and brown for 2 min.

2. Add the previously floured and salted pork slices (directly over the chicory), simmer for 6 minutes turning them over after 3 minutes.

3. Remove the slices and place them on a serving plate, covering them with the rest of the red chicory juice collected at the bottom of the basket.

Nutrition:

☐ Calories 504 ☐ Fat 33 ☐ Carbohydrates 0g

☐ Sugars 0g ☐ Protein 42g

☐ Cholesterol 130mg

Pork and Parsni With Thai, Marinated with Honey and Soy

Preparation Time: 20 minutes;

Cooking time: 30 minutes;

Serving: 2

Ingredients:

- ★ ☐ 2 pork ribs to choose from the tenderloin

- ★ ☐ 1 large parsnip

- ★ ☐ 1 coriander leaf

- ★ ☐ 1 sprig fresh chopped parsley

- ★ ☐ Salt

- ★ ☐ For the marinade:

- ★ ☐ 2 tbsp olive oil

- ★ ☐ 2 tbsp soy sauce

- ★ ☐ The juice of half a lemon

- ★ ☐ 1 tbsp of honey, preferably flavored with orange blossom

- ★ ☐ 1 tsp of specific spices for wok Preparation Time

- ★ ☐ 1 tsp of Asian spice mix

- ★ ☐ Coriander powder

Direction:

1. Preparation Timeare the marinade by mixing all the ingredients in a large bowl. Mix to obtain a very homogeneous mixture.

2. Dip the pork chunks in the marinade, turning them over to make sure it covers the meat ribs perfectly. Preparation Timeare the parsnip by peeling and washing it, and then cut it into small dice.

3. Use a large plate to place the pieces of pork and parsnips covered with marinade. Pour the parsnips into the bowl and mix. Let stand for at least 1 hour before cooking.

4. Set the air fryer at 1600C without oil for 30 minutes and cook the parsnips.

5. At the end of the 10 minutes of cooking, add the pieces of pork or proceed to a traditional baking in the oven with 10 minutes on each side being careful to keep the cooking juices.

Nutrition:

☐ Calories 179

☐ Carbohydrates 11g

☐ Fat 13g

☐ Sugars 6g

☐ Protein 1g

☐ Cholesterol 0mg

Pork Fillet Mignon

Preparation Time: 5 minutes;

Cooking time: 12 minutes;

Serving: 3

Ingredients:

★ ☐ 6 medallions of 100g to 150g cut in a pork loin

★ ☐ Olive oil

★ ☐ Salt and pepper

Direction:

1. Cut six pork medallions the same size as the pork loin you own.

2. Salt and pepper to your liking.

3. Use a cooking tool to spray a very small amount of olive oil.

4. Place your pork medallions on the air fryer previously preheated at 1500C and cook for 12 minutes.

Nutrition:

☐ Calories 125

☐ Fat 3.4g

☐ Carbohydrates 0g

☐ Sugars 0g

☐ Protein 22g ☐ Cholesterol 62mg

Taco Stuffed Peppers

Preparation Time: 10 minutes

Cooking Time: 15 minutes

Servings: 4

Ingredients:

- ☐ 1 lb. ground beef

- ☐ 1 tbsp. taco seasoning mix ☐ 1 can diced tomatoes and green chilis

- ☐ 4 green bell peppers ☐ 1 cup shredded Monterey jack cheese, divided

Directions:

1. Set a skillet over a high heat and cook the ground beef for seven to ten minutes. Make sure it is cooked through and brown all over. Drain the fat.

2. Stir in the taco seasoning mix, as well as the diced tomatoes and green chilis. Allow the mixture to cook for a further three to five minutes.

3. In the meantime, slice the tops off the green peppers and remove the seeds and membranes.

4. When the meat mixture is fully cooked, spoon equal amounts of it into the peppers and top with the Monterey jack cheese. Then place the peppers into your fryer.

5. Cook at 350°F for fifteen minutes.

6. The peppers are ready when they are soft and the cheese is bubbling and brown. Serve warm and enjoy!

Nutrition: Calories: 282, Fats: 19.9g, Carbohydrates: 6.6g, Sugar: 5.9g,

Proteins: 18.4g, Sodium: 357mg

Beef Tenderloin & Peppercorn Crust

Preparation Time: 10 minutes

Cooking Time: 25 minutes

Servings: 4

Ingredients:

★ ☐ 2 lb. beef tenderloin

★ ☐ 2 tsp. roasted garlic, minced

★ ☐ 2 tbsp. salted butter, melted

★ ☐ 3 tbsp. ground 4-peppercorn blender

Directions:

1. Remove any surplus fat from the beef tenderloin.

2. Combine the roasted garlic and melted butter to apply to your tenderloin with a brush.

3. On a plate, spread out the peppercorns and roll the tenderloin in them, making sure they are covering and clinging to the meat.

4. Cook the tenderloin in your fryer for twenty-five minutes at 400°F, turning halfway through cooking.

5. Let the tenderloin rest for ten minutes before slicing and serving.

Nutrition:

Calories: 433,

Fats: 19.9g,

Carbohydrates: 4.6g, Sugar: 6.9g, Proteins: 48.4g, Sodium: 237mg

Bratwursts

Preparation Time: 10 minutes

Cooking Time: 25 minutes

Servings: 1

Ingredients:

★ □ 4 x 3-oz. beef bratwursts

Directions:

1. Place the beef bratwursts in the basket of your fryer and cook for fifteen minutes at 375°F, turning once halfway through.

2. Enjoy with the low-carb toppings and sides of your choice.

Nutrition:

Calories: 32,

Fats: 23.9g,

Carbohydrates: 12.6g,

Sugar: 5.9g,

Proteins: 38.4g,

Sodium: 237mg

Bacon-Wrapped Hot Dog

Preparation Time: 5 minutes

Cooking Time: 10 minutes

Servings: 4

Ingredients:

★ ☐ 4 slices sugar-free bacon

★ ☐ 4 beef hot dogs

Directions:

1. Take a slice of bacon and wrap it around the hot dog, securing it with a toothpick. Repeat with the other pieces of bacon and hot dogs, placing each wrapped dog in the basket of your fryer.

2. Cook at 370°F for ten minutes, turning halfway through to fry the other side.

3. Once hot and crispy, the hot dogs are ready to serve. Enjoy!

Nutrition:

Calories: 282,

Fats: 19.9g,

Carbohydrates: 6.6g,

Sugar: 5.9g,

Proteins: 18.4g,

Sodium: 357mg

Herb Shredded Beef

Preparation Time: 10 minutes

Cooking Time: 20 minutes

Servings: 1

Ingredients:

★ ☐ 1 tsp. dried dill

★ ☐ 1 tsp. dried thyme

★ ☐ 1 tsp. garlic powder

★ ☐ 2 lbs. beefsteak

★ ☐ 3 tbsp. butter

Directions:

1. Pre-heat your fryer at 360°F.

2. Combine the dill, thyme, and garlic powder together, and massage into the steak.

3. Cook the steak in the fryer for twenty minutes, then remove, shred, and return to the fryer. Add the butter and cook for a further two minutes at 365°F. Make sure the beef is coated in the butter before serving.

Nutrition:

Calories: 444,

Fats: 19.9g,

Carbohydrates: 6.6g,

Sugar: 5.9g, Proteins: 28.4g, Sodium: 57mg

Herbed Butter Rib Eye Steak

Preparation Time: 10 minutes

Cooking Time: 30 minutes

Servings: 2

Ingredients:

- ★ ☐ 4 ribeye steaks

- ★ ☐ Olive oil

- ★ ☐ ¾ tsp. dry rub

- ★ ☐ ½ cup butter

- ★ ☐ 1 tsp. dried basil

- ★ ☐ 3 tbsp. lemon garlic seasoning

Directions:

1. Massage the olive oil into the steaks and your favorite dry rub. Leave aside to sit for thirty minutes.

2. In a bowl, combine the button, dried basil, and lemon garlic seasoning, then refrigerate.

3. Pre-heat the fryer at 450°F and set a rack inside. Place the steaks on top of the rack and allow to cook for fifteen minutes.

4. Remove the steaks from the fryer when cooked and serve with the herbed butter.

Nutrition:

Calories: 232,

Fats: 11.9g, Carbohydrates: 8.6g, Sugar: 8.9g, Proteins: 23.4g, Sodium: 227mg

Flank Steak & Avocado Butter

Preparation Time: 5 minutes

Cooking Time: 15 minutes

Servings: 4

Ingredients:

★ ☐ 1 flank steak

★ ☐ Salt and pepper

★ ☐ 2 avocados

★ ☐ 2 tbsp. butter, melted

★ ☐ ½ cup chimichurri sauce

Directions:

1. Rub the flank steak with salt and pepper to taste and leave to sit for twenty minutes.

2. Pre-heat the fryer at 400°F and place a rack inside.

3. Halve the avocados and take out the pits. Spoon the flesh into a bowl and mash with a fork. Mix in the melted butter and chimichurri sauce, making sure everything is well combined.

4. Put the steak in the fryer and cook for six minutes. Flip over and allow to cook for another six minutes.

5. Serve the steak with the avocado butter and enjoy!

Nutrition: Calories: 322, Fats: 19.9g, Carbohydrates: 6.6g, Sugar: 2.9g,

Proteins: 18.4g,

Sodium: 300mg

Preparation Time: 15 minutes

Cooking Time: 25 minutes

Servings: 2

Ingredients:

★ ☐ 1 tbsp. butter, melted

★ ☐ ¼ dried thyme

★ ☐ 1 tsp. garlic salt

★ ☐ ¼ tsp. dried parsley

★ ☐ 1 lb. beef loin

Directions:

1. In a bowl, combine the melted butter, thyme, garlic salt, and parsley.

2. Cut the beef loin into slices and generously apply the seasoned butter using a brush.

3. Pre-heat your fryer at 400°F and place a rack inside.

4. Cook the beef for fifteen minutes.

5. Take care when removing it, and serve hot.

Nutrition:

Calories: 322,

Fats: 29.9g,

Carbohydrates: 15.6g,

Sugar: 11.9g, Proteins: 11.4g, Sodium: 357mg

Lamb Ribs

Preparation Time: 10 minutes

Cooking Time: 25 minutes

Servings: 1

Ingredients:

★ ☐ 1 lb. lamb ribs

★ ☐ 2 tbsp. mustard

★ ☐ 1 tsp. rosemary, chopped

★ ☐ Salt and pepper

★ ☐ ¼ cup mint leaves, chopped

★ ☐ 1 cup Green yogurt

Directions:

1. Pre-heat the fryer at 350°F.

2. Use a brush to apply the mustard to the lamb ribs, and season with rosemary, as well as salt and pepper as desired.

3. Cook the ribs in the fryer for eighteen minutes.

4. Meanwhile, combine together the mint leaves and yogurt in a bowl.

5. Remove the lamb ribs from the fryer when cooked and serve with the mint yogurt. Enjoy!

Nutrition: Calories: 333, Fats: 13.9g, Carbohydrates: 2.6g, Sugar: 7.9g, Proteins: 32.4g,

Sodium: 437mg

Lamb Satay

Preparation Time: 15 minutes

Cooking Time: 20 minutes

Servings: 3

Ingredients:

- ★ ☐ ¼ tsp. cumin

- ★ ☐ 1 tsp ginger

- ★ ☐ ½ tsp. nutmeg

- ★ ☐ Salt and pepper

- ★ ☐ 2 boneless lamb steaks

- ★ ☐ Olive oil cooking spray

Directions:

1. Combine the cumin, ginger, nutmeg, salt and pepper in a bowl.

2. Cube the lamb steaks and massage the spice mixture into each one.

3. Leave to marinate for ten minutes, then transfer onto metal skewers.

4. Pre-heat the fryer at 400°F.

5. Spritz the skewers with the olive oil cooking spray, then cook them in the fryer for eight minutes.

6. Take care when removing them from the fryer, and serve with the low-carb sauce of your choice.

Nutrition:

Calories: 282, Fats: 19.9g, Carbohydrates: 6.6g, Sugar: 5.9g, Proteins: 18.4g, Sodium: 357mg

ITALIAN RECIPES

Italian Lamb Chops

Preparation Time: 10 minutes

Cooking Time: 30 minutes

Servings: 1

Ingredients:

- ★ ☐ 2 lamp chops

- ★ ☐ 2 tsp. Italian herbs

- ★ ☐ 2 avocados

- ★ ☐ ½ cup mayonnaise

- ★ ☐ 1 tbsp. lemon juice

Directions:

1. Season the lamb chops with the Italian herbs, then set aside for five minutes.

2. Pre-heat the fryer at 400°F and place the rack inside.

3. Put the chops on the rack and allow to cook for twelve minutes.

4. In the meantime, halve the avocados and open to remove the pits. Spoon the flesh into a blender.

5. Add in the mayonnaise and lemon juice and pulse until a smooth consistency is achieved.

6. Take care when removing the chops from the fryer, then plate up and serve with the avocado mayo.

Nutrition: Calories: 332, Fats: 19.9g, Carbohydrates: 4.6g, S Sugar: 5.9g, Proteins: 38.4g, Sodium: 127mg

Simple Basil Tomatoes

Preparation Time: 10 minutes

Cooking Time: 10 minutes

Servings: 2

Ingredients:

☐ 3 tomatoes

☐ Olive oil cooking spray

☐ Salt and pepper to taste

☐ 1 tablespoon fresh basil, chopped

Directions:

1. Cut tomatoes in halves and drizzle them well with cooking spray

2. Sprinkle salt, pepper, and basil

3. Press "Power Button" on your Air Fryer and select "Air Fry" mode

4. Press the Time Button and set time to 20 minutes

5. Push Temp Button and set temp to 320 degrees F

6. Press the "Start/Pause" button and start the device

7. Once the appliance beeps to indicated that it is pre-heated, arrange tomatoes in Air Fryer cooking basket, let them cook

8. Once done, serve warm and enjoy!

Nutrition:: Calories: 34 Fat: 0.4 g Saturated Fat: 0.1 g Carbohydrates: 7 g Fiber: 2 g ☐ ☐ Sodium: 87 mg ☐ Protein: 1.7 g

Parm Asparagus

Preparation Time: 10 minutes

Cooking Time: 10 minutes

Servings: 3

Ingredients: ☐ 1-pound asparagus, trimmed

☐ 1 tablespoon parmesan cheese, grated ☐ 1 tablespoon butter, melted

☐ 1 teaspoon garlic powder ☐ Salt and pepper to taste

Directions:

1. Take a bowl and add asparagus, cheese, butter, garlic powder, salt, and pepper

2. Press "Power Button" on your Air Fryer and select "Air Fry" mode

3. Press the Time Button and set time to 10 minutes

4. Push Temp Button and set temp to 400 degrees F

5. Press the "Start/Pause" button and start the device

6. Once the appliance beeps to indicated that it is pre-heated, arrange the vegetable mixture in Air Fryer cooking basket, let them cook

7. Once done, serve warm and enjoy!

Nutrition:: ☐ Calories: 70 Fat: 4 g Saturated Fat: 2 g Carbohydrates: 6 g

☐ Fiber: 3 g

☐ Sodium: 96 mg

☐ Protein: 4 g

Spiced Up Butternut Squash

Preparation Time: 15 minutes

Cooking Time: 20 minutes

Servings: 4

Ingredients:

☐ 1 medium butternut squash, peeled, seeded and cut into chunks

☐ 2 teaspoons cumin seeds ☐ 1/8 teaspoon garlic powder

☐ 1/98 teaspoon chili flakes, crushed ☐ Salt and pepper to taste

☐ 1 tablespoon pine nuts ☐ 2 tablespoons fresh cilantro

Directions:

1. Take a bowl and add squash, spices, and oil

2. Press "Power Button" on your Air Fryer and select "Air Fry" mode

3. Press the Time Button and set time to 20 minutes

4. Push Temp Button and set temp to 375 degrees F

5. Press the "Start/Pause" button and start the device

6. Arrange squash chunks into your Air Fryer cooking basket and push into oven

7. Let it cook until done, serve with a sprinkle of cilantro and pine nuts

8. Enjoy!

Nutrition:: ☐ Calories: 190 ☐ Fat: 7 g ☐ Saturated Fat: 0.8 g ☐ Carbohydrates: 34 g ☐ Fiber: 6 g ☐ Sodium: 53 mg ☐ Protein: 3 g

Hearty Caramelized Baby Carrots

Preparation Time: 10 minutes

Cooking Time: 15 minutes

Servings: 4

Ingredients:

☐ ½ cup butter, melted

☐ ½ cup brown sugar

☐ A 1-pound bag of baby carrots

Directions:

1. Take a bowl and mix in brown sugar, butter, and carrots

2. Press "Power Button" on your Air Fryer and select "Air Fry" mode

3. Press the Time Button and set time to 15 minutes

4. Push Temp Button and set temp to 400 degrees F

5. Press the "Start/Pause" button and start the device

6. Arrange carrots int the cooking basket (greased), let it cook until the timer runs out

7. Serve and enjoy!

Nutrition::

☐ Calories: 3120 ☐ Fat: 23 g ☐ Saturated Fat: 14 g ☐ Carbohydrates: 27 g

☐ Fiber: 3 g ☐ Sodium: 257 mg

☐ Protein: 1 g

Sweet Potatoes And Broccoli

Preparation Time: 15 minutes

Cooking Time: 20 minutes

Servings: 4

Ingredients:

☐ 2 medium sweet potatoes, peeled and cut into 1-inch cubes

☐ 1 head broccoli, cut into 1-inch florets

☐ 2 tablespoons vegetable oil

☐ Salt and pepper to taste

Directions:

1. Take a large-sized bowl and add all listed ingredients

2. Toss them well to coat them

3. Press "Power Button" on your Air Fryer and select "Air Roast" mode

4. Press the Time Button and set time to 20 minutes

5. Push Temp Button and set temp to 415 degrees F

6. Press the "Start/Pause" button and start the device

7. Arrange prepared carrots to cooking basket (greased)

8. Push it in and let it cook until the timer runs out

9. Take a large-sized bowl and add remaining butter, zucchini, basil, salt, and pepper, mix well

10. After the first 5 minutes of cooking, pour the zucchini mixture into the cooking basket alongside carrots

11. Let it cook

12. Serve and enjoy!

Nutrition:: ☐ Calories: 170 ☐ Fat: 8 g ☐ Saturated Fat: 1.4 g ☐ Carbohydrates: 25 g ☐ Fiber: 4 g ☐ Sodium: 67 mg ☐ Protein: 3 g

Cauliflower And Broccoli Dish

Preparation Time: 15 minutes

Cooking Time: 20 minutes

Servings: 4

Ingredients:

☐ 1 and ½ cups broccoli, cut into 1-inch pieces

☐ 1 and ½ cups cauliflower, cut into 1-inch pieces

☐ 1 tablespoon olive oil

☐ Salt as needed

Directions:

1. Take a bowl and add vegetables, oil, and salt. Toss well and coat them well

2. Press "Power Button" on your Air Fryer and select "Air Fry" mode

3. Press the Time Button and set time to 20 minutes

4. Push Temp Button and set temp to 375 degrees F

5. Press the "Start/Pause" button and start the device

6. Arrange the vegetable mixture into your Air Fryer Basket and push it into the oven, let it cook until the timer runs out

7. Serve and enjoy!

Nutrition:: ☐ Calories: 60 ☐ Fat: 4 g ☐ Saturated Fat: 0.5 g ☐ Carbohydrates: 4 g ☐ Fiber: 2 g ☐ Sodium: 61 mg ☐ Protein: 2 g

Hearty Lemon Green Beans

Preparation Time: 15 minutes

Cooking Time: 12 minutes

Servings: 4

Ingredients:

☐ 1-pound green beans, trimmed

☐ 1 tablespoon butter, melted

☐ 1 tablespoon fresh lemon juice

☐ ¼ teaspoon garlic powder

☐ Salt and pepper to taste

☐ ½ teaspoon lemon zest, grated

Directions:

1. Take a large-sized bowl and add all listed ingredients, except lemon zest

2. Toss and coat well

3. Press "Power Button" on your Air Fryer and select "Air Fry" mode

4. Press the Time Button and set time to 12 minutes

5. Push Temp Button and set temp to 400 degrees F

6. Press the "Start/Pause" button and start the device

7. Arrange the green beans into Air Fryer basket and push into the oven, let it cook until the timer runs out

8. Serve warm with a garnish with lemon zest!

Nutrition::

☐ Calories: 60

☐ Fat: 3 g

☐ Saturated Fat: 1.9 g

☐ Carbohydrates: 8 g

☐ Fiber: 3 g

☐ Sodium: 67 mg

☐ Protein: 2 g

Green Beans With Okra

Preparation Time: 15 minutes

Cooking Time: 20 minutes

Servings: 2

Ingredients:

☐ 10 ounces frozen cut okra

☐ 10 ounces frozen green beans

☐ ¼ cup Nutrition:al yeast

☐ 3 tablespoons balsamic vinegar ☐ Salt and pepper to taste

Directions:

1. Take a bowl and add okra, green beans, Nutrition:al yeast, vinegar, salt, pepper and toss the mixture well, make sure everything is coated well

2. Press "Power Button" on your Air Fryer and select "Air Fry" mode

3. Press the Time Button and set time to 20 minutes

4. Push Temp Button and set temp to 400 degrees F

5. Press the "Start/Pause" button and start the device

6. Grease the Air Fryer basket well and arrange okra mixture in the basket

7. Put the basket in the oven and let it cook, until it Is done

8. Enjoy!

Nutrition:: ☐ Calories: 125 ☐ Fat: 2 g ☐ Saturated Fat: 0.2 g ☐ Carbohydrates: 19 g ☐ Fiber: 10 g ☐ Sodium: 100 mg ☐ Protein: 11 g

Glazed Mushrooms

Preparation Time: 10 minutes

Cooking Time: 15 minutes

Servings: 4

Ingredients: □ ½ cup low-sodium soy sauce □ 2 teaspoons honey

□ 4 tablespoons balsamic vinegar □ 2 teaspoons Chinese Five-Spice powder

□ ½ teaspoon ground ginger □ 20 ounces fresh cremini mushrooms, halved

Directions:

1. Take a bowl and add soy sauce, honey, garlic, vinegar, five-spice powder, ground ginger and mix well

2. Arrange mushroom mixture in a greased-up baking pan in a single layer

3. Press "Power Button" on your Air Fryer and select "Air Fry" mode

4. Press the Time Button and set time to 15 minutes

5. Push Temp Button and set temp to 350 degrees F

6. Press the "Start/Pause" button and start the device

7. Arrange the pan over a wire rack and insert in the oven, let it cook for 10 minutes, add vinegar mixture on top

8. Stir well, let it cook until done

9. Serve and enjoy!

Nutrition:: □ Calories: 54 □ Fat: 0.1 g □ Saturated Fat: 0 g □ Carbohydrates: 9.6 g □ Fiber: 0.8 g □ Sodium: 1400 mg □ Protein: 4 g

Herbed Bell Pepper

Preparation Time: 10 minutes

Cooking Time: 8 minutes

Servings: 4

Ingredients:

☐ 1 and ½ pounds bell pepper, seeded and cubed

☐ ½ teaspoon dried thyme, crushed ☐ ½ teaspoon dried savory, crushed

☐ Salt and pepper to taste ☐ 2 teaspoons butter, melted

Directions:

1. Take a bowl and add bell pepper herbs, salt, pepper and toss well

2. Press "Power Button" on your Air Fryer and select "Air Fry" mode

3. Press the Time Button and set time to 8 minutes

4. Push Temp Button and set temp to 360 degrees F

5. Press the "Start/Pause" button and start the device

6. Arrange bell pepper in the Air Fryer basket and push it in the oven

7. Drizzle with butter, let it cook until done

8. Serve and enjoy!

Nutrition:: ☐ Calories: 32 ☐ Fat: 2 g ☐ Saturated Fat: 1.2 g ☐ Carbohydrates: 4 g ☐ Fiber: 0.7 g ☐ Sodium: 54 mg ☐ Protein: 0.5 g

BEEF RECIPES

Mozzarella Beef

Preparation Time: 10

Cooking Time: 15

Servings: 1

Ingredients:

- ★ ☐ 12 oz. beef brisket

- ★ ☐ 2 tsp. Italian herbs

- ★ ☐ 2 tsp. butter

- ★ ☐ 1 onion, sliced

- ★ ☐ 7 oz. mozzarella cheese, sliced

Directions:

1. Pre-heat the fryer at 365°F.

2. Cut up the brisket into four equal slices and season with the Italian herbs.

3. Allow the butter to melt in the fryer. Place the slices of beef inside along with the onion. Put a piece of mozzarella on top of each piece of brisket, and cook for twenty-five minutes.

Enjoy!

Nutrition: Calories: 382, Fats: 19.9g, Carbohydrates: 9.6g, Sugar: 2.9g, Proteins: 18.4g, Sodium: 221mg

Rosemary Rib Eye Steaks

Preparation Time: 15 minutes

Cooking Time: 20 minutes

Servings: 1

Ingredients:

- ★ ☐ ¼ cup butter

- ★ ☐ 1 clove minced garlic

- ★ ☐ Salt and pepper

- ★ ☐ 1 ½ tbsp. balsamic vinegar

- ★ ☐ ¼ cup rosemary, chopped

- ★ ☐ 2 ribeye steaks

Directions:

1. Melt the butter in a skillet over medium heat. Add the garlic and fry until fragrant.

2. Remove the skillet from the heat and add in the salt, pepper, and vinegar. Allow it to cool.

3. Add the rosemary, then pour the whole mixture into a Ziploc bag.

4. Put the ribeye steaks in the bag and shake well, making sure to coat the meat well. Refrigerate for an hour, then allow to sit for a further twenty minutes.

5. Pre-heat the fryer at 400°F and set the rack inside. Cook the ribeyes for fifteen minutes.

6. Take care when removing the steaks from the fryer and plate up. Enjoy!

Nutrition: Calories: 444, Fats: 19.9g, Carbohydrates: 8.6g, Sugar: 9.9g, Proteins: 23.4g, S Sodium: 231mg

Meatloaf

Preparation Time: 10

Cooking Time: 15

Servings: 4

Ingredients:

☐ 1 egg

☐ 1 lb. ground beef

☐ 1 cup cheddar cheese, shredded

☐ ¼ cup chopped onion

☐ ½ cup tomato purée

Directions:

1. Break the egg into a bowl, add desired seasoning, and whisk well with a fork.

2. Add the ground beef, cheese, and onion to the bowl, combining everything with your hands to make sure everything is well-incorporated.

3. Put the mixture in a silicon loaf pan, pressing down on the top to ensure it is even. Pour the tomato purée over the top, then set the pan aside.

4. Pre-heat the fryer at 350°F. Cook the mixture for twenty minutes.

5. Take care when taking the pan out of the fryer, and let it cool for a few minutes before serving.

Nutrition:

Calories: 382, Fats: 29.9g, Carbohydrates: 7.6g, Sugar: 8.9g, Proteins: 48.4g, Sodium: 327mg

Perfect Garlic Butter Steak

Preparation Time: 20 min.

Cooking time: 12 min.

Serving: 1

Ingredients:

★ ☐ 2 Ribeye steaks

★ ☐ Salt

★ ☐ Pepper

★ ☐ Olive oil

★ ☐ Garlic butter:

★ ☐ ½ cup softened butter

★ ☐ 2 tbsp chopped fresh parsley

★ ☐ 2 garlic cloves, minced

★ ☐ 1 tsp Worcestershire sauce

★ ☐ ½ tsp salt (optional)

Direction:

1. Preparation Time are the garlic butter by mixing all the ingredients together.

2. Place in parchment paper. Roll up and put in the fridge.

3. Let the steaks sit for 20 minutes at room temperature.

4. Brush with a little oil, salt, and pepper.

5. Preheat your hot air fryer to 400°F (200°C).

6. Cook for 12 minutes, turning halfway through cooking. Serve.

7. Place the garlic butter on the steaks and let sit for 5 minutes.

8. Enjoy!

Nutrition: Calories 250 ☐ Fat 10g ☐ Carbohydrates 2g ☐ Sugars 1g ☐ Protein 36g ☐ Cholesterol 100mg

Crispy Pork Medallions

Preparation Time: 20 minutes;

Cooking time: 5 minutes;

Serving: 2

Ingredients:

☐ 1 pork loin, 330 g, cut into 6 or 7 slices of 4 cm

☐ 1 tsp Dijon mustard

☐ 1 tsp oil

☐ Salt, pepper and paprika

☐ Asian marinade

☐ 1 tsp salt reduced tamari sauce

☐ 1 tsp olive oil

☐ 1 clementine juice

☐ 1 pinch cayenne pepper

☐ 2 cloves garlic, pressed

☐ Crunchy coating

☐ 1/3 cup breadcrumbs

☐ ½ orange zest

☐ 2g freshly grated Parmesan cheese

Direction:

1. Preparation Time are the marinade first. In a bowl, combine all the ingredients. Lightly salt the medallions, pepper, and sprinkle with paprika. Place these in the marinade and turn them several times to impregnate them completely. Cover with plastic wrap and marinate for 1 hour at room temperature.

2. Preparation Time are the coating by combining the breadcrumbs, the orange zest, and the Parmesan cheese in a deep dish.

3. When the maceration time has elapsed, remove the marinade medallions, and dry them on absorbent paper. Spread with mustard, then move on to the crunchy layer. Brush lightly with oil.

4. Heat the air fryer to 350°F. Place the medallions in the fryer basket. Cook 5 minutes, stir, and then return to the fryer for another minute. Serve immediately.

Nutrition:

☐ Calories 222

☐ Carbohydrates 13g

☐ Fat 6g

☐ Protein 24g ☐ Sugars 0h ☐ Cholesterol 74mg

Nemos Beef with Dry Pepper Lactose Free

Preparation Time: 30 minutes;

Cooking time: 20-25 minutes;

Serving: 5

Ingredients:

- ★ ☐ 250g of minced meat

- ★ ☐ 1 handful of rice noodles

- ★ ☐ 25 rice leaves

- ★ ☐ 1 small onion

- ★ ☐ 1 clove garlic

- ★ ☐ 1 cube of chicken broth

- ★ ☐ Roasted Sesame Oil

- ★ ☐ 2 tsp dried pepper

- ★ ☐ 1 tbsp soy sauce

- ★ ☐ 1 tsp ground ginger

Direction:

1. Finely chop the onion and garlic and mix with the minced meat. Add half of the dried pepper, being careful to crush it beforehand. Add the ginger powder and soy sauce. Brown the Preparation Time in roasted sesame oil, making sure you only have small pieces of minced meat.

2. Bring a pan of boiling water to which you will add chicken broth. Dip the rice noodles in it for only 3 minutes.

3. Add them to the ground beef Preparation Time and then add the rest of the dried pepper.

4. Lightly moisten the rice leaves, place the filling in the middle and close them to create a perfect nem.

5. Place the spring rolls in the air fryer without oil previously heated at 1500C and cook for 10 to 15 minutes, according to taste.

Nutrition:

☐ Calories 203

☐ Carbohydrates 7g

☐ Fat 15g

☐ Protein 12g

☐ Sugars 5g

☐ Cholesterol 0mg

Lamb with Potatoes

Preparation Time: 10-20 minutes;

Cooking time: 30 - 45 minutes;

Serving: 2

Ingredients:

- ☐ 1 kg Lamb milk in pieces ☐ 600g Fresh potatoes

- ☐ 5 spoons Sunflower oil

- ☐ Salt and pepper

- ☐ 2 spoons Sage, rosemary, thyme

- ☐ ½ glass White wine

Direction:

1. Remove the mixing paddle from the tank.

2. Put the pieces of lamb, oil, sage, rosemary, and thyme in the cooking pot. Close the cover, set the thermostat to position 4, press the lower resistance power key and press the on / off key; brown for 4 min.

3. Add the wine and simmer for another 6 min.

4. Preheat the air fryer at 1500C for 5 minutes.

5. Finally pour the potatoes cut into pieces, salt, pepper and cook for 35 min. Extra by mixing the potatoes manually 2-3 times during cooking.

Nutrition: ☐ Calories 372.0 ☐ Fat 12.3 g ☐ Carbohydrate 34.1 g ☐ Sugars1.9 ☐ Protein31.5 g ☐ Cholesterol 86.7 mg

Veal Blanquette With Peas

Preparation Time: 10-20;

Cooking time: 45-60;

Serving: 2

Ingredients:

★ □ 600g Veal meat

★ □ 250g Frozen peas

★ □ ½ Onions

★ □ ½ glass White wine

★ □ 1 tsp Oil

★ □ 250 ml Broth

Direction:

1. Chop the onion and put it inside the tank with the oil. Close the lid

2. Brown for 5 min setting the air fryer at 1500C.

3. Add lightly floured meat, white wine, and simmer for 10 minutes.

4. Then add frozen peas, broth, salt, pepper, and simmer for 35 minutes. additional depending on the desired degree of cooking.

Nutrition:

□ Calories 418□ Carbohydrates 24g □ Fat 14g □ Sugars 0g □ Protein 49g □ Cholesterol 357mg

Beef Stroganoff

Preparation Time: 10-20;

Cooking time: 15 – 30;

Serving: 6

Ingredients:

- ☐ 1000 g beef ☐ 500g onion
- ☐ Mushrooms 500g ☐ 150g sour cream
- ☐ 50 g butter ☐ 100 g of broth
- ☐ Salt, pepper to taste
- ☐ 2 tbsp paprika
- ☐ Flour

Direction:

1. Cut the onion into very thin slices, then clean the mushrooms well and cut them into slices, finally cut the meat into strips about 5 cm long.

2. Place the butter, onion, and mushrooms on the baking sheet.

3. Preheat the air fryer at 200C for 5 minutes. Simmer for 10 min.

4. Add the floured meat, paprika, broth, salt, pepper, and simmer for another 10 minutes.

5. Finally pour the cream and finish cooking for another 5 minutes or until ready.

Nutrition:

Calories 391 ☐ Fat 23g ☐ Carbohydrates 21g ☐ Sugars 3.2g ☐ Protein 25g☐ Cholesterol 115mg

Meatballs with Tomatoes and Peas

Preparation Time: 10 – 20;

Cooking time: 15 - 30,

Serving: 6

Ingredients:

★ ☐ 425 g minced meat

★ ☐ 1 egg

★ ☐ 25 g grated cheese

★ ☐ Salt to taste

★ ☐ To taste breadcrumbs

★ ☐ Parsley chopped to taste

★ ☐ 150 g of frozen peas

★ ☐ 400 g of tomatoes cut into large pieces

★ ☐ 1 tsp oil

★ ☐ 2 shallots

Direction:

1. Put the minced meat, the egg, the grated cheese, the salt, the parsley, the breadcrumbs in a bowl and mix until you get a consistent mixture. Form the meatballs (with these doses you will get 15-18 meatballs).

2. Chop the shallots and pour them into the basket greased with the oil. Close. Set the air fryer at 1500C and brown for 3 min.

3. Add the meatballs and simmer for an additional 7 minutes.

4. Then add the frozen peas, tomato, salt and pepper and simmer for another 18 minutes.

Nutrition:

☐ Calories 40

☐ Fat 2.9 g

☐ Carbohydrates 0.9 g

☐ Sugars0.5 g

☐ Protein 2.7 g

☐ Cholesterol 15 mg

Cevapi

Preparation Time: more than 30;

Cooking time: 15 – 30;

Serving: 4

Ingredients:

★ ☐ 150g of onion

★ ☐ 350g ground beef

★ ☐ 150g minced pork

★ ☐ Leave at discretion

★ ☐ Pepper at discretion

★ ☐ Red paprika at discretion

Direction:

1. Mix all the ingredients in a bowl (the onion must be finely chopped) and knead well; form rolls 4 to 5 cm long and let stand in the refrigerator for at least 1 hour.

2. Place the cevapi in the basket of the air fryer. Set the temperature to 1500C.

3. Cook the cevapis (8 at a time) for about 13 to 15 minutes, turning them in the middle of cooking.

Nutrition: ☐ Calories 63 ☐ Fat 4.84g ☐ Carbohydrates 0.25g ☐ Sugars 0.02g ☐ Protein 4.19g ☐ Cholesterol 17mg

Milanese Chop

Preparation Time: 10 – 20;

Cooking time: 15 – 30;

Serving: 2

Ingredients:

★ ☐ 2 veal chops

★ ☐ 1 egg

★ ☐ 70 g of breadcrumbs

★ ☐ Salt to taste

★ ☐ 1 tsp oil

Direction:

1. Beat the egg in a bowl and Preparation Timeare the breadcrumbs on a flat plate.

2. Pass each chop in the egg and then in breadcrumbs. Press the meat firmly into the pie. Put in the refrigerator for at least half an hour.

3. Pour the oil into the basket. Place the two chops.

4. Set the air fryer to 1500 and cook the meat for 10 minutes and then turn the chop.

5. Cook for 5 minutes additional.

6. Serve the chops still hot, covering the bone with aluminum foil to facilitate tasting.

Nutrition:

☐ Calories 231

☐ Carbohydrates 8g

☐ Fat 9g

☐ Sugars 0g

☐ Protein 27g

☐ Cholesterol 97mg

Lemon Chops

Preparation Time: 0-10;

Cooking time: 0-15;

Serving: 2

Ingredients:

★ ☐ 4 slices of pork

★ ☐ 40g butter

★ ☐ Flour to taste

★ ☐ 1 lemon juice

★ ☐ Salt to taste

Direction:

1. Preheat the air fryer at 1800C for 5 minutes.

2. Flour the pork slices. Place the butter in the basket and brown for 2 minutes.

3. Add the previously floured and salted pork slices, simmer for 3 another minutes. Turn them on themselves.

4. Add the lemon juice and simmer for 3 another minutes.

5. Remove the slices and add a pinch of butter to the tank to thicken the juice. Mix the juice with a wooden spoon and pour the scallops over it.

6. Serve decorating the dish with lemon julienne.

Nutrition: ☐ Calories 242.4 ☐ Fat 15.7 g ☐ Carbohydrate 0.7 g ☐ Sugars 0.0 g ☐ Protein 23.2 g ☐ Cholesterol 65.9 mg

Amatriciana

Preparation Time: 0-10 minutes;

Cooking time: 15-30 minutes;

Serving: 4

Ingredients:

★ □ 200g Pork cheek

★ □ 1 Medium onion

★ □ 400g Peeled tomatoes

★ □ 3 spoons Oil

★ □ 1 Chile

★ □ Salt

Direction:

1. Chop the onion and cut the pork cheek (removing the hard shell). Put everything in the basket, adding the oil.

2. Close the cover, set the air fryer to 3 minutes at 1500C to brown. Then pour the tomato, pepper, and salt.

3. Cook for an additional 17 minutes, or until desired cooking is achieved.

Nutrition:

□ Calories 321 □ Fat 9g □ Carbohydrate 49g □ Sugars 50g □ Protein 14g □ Cholesterol 20mg

Venetian Liver

Preparation Time: 10-20;

Cooking time: 15-30;

Serving: 6

Ingredients:

★ ☐ 500g veal liver

★ ☐ 2 white onions

★ ☐ 100g of water

★ ☐ 2 tbsp vinegar

★ ☐ Salt and pepper to taste

Direction:

1. Chop the onion and put it inside the pan with the water. Set the air fryer to 1800C and cook for 20 minutes.

2. Add the liver cut into small pieces and vinegar, close the lid, and cook for an additional 10 minutes.

3. Add salt and pepper.

Nutrition:

☐ Calories 131

☐ Fat 14.19 g ☐ Carbohydrates 16.40 g

☐ Sugars 5.15 g

☐ Protein 25.39 g ☐ Cholesterol 350.41 mg

VEGETABLE RECIPES

Creamy Beets

Preparation time: 5 minutes

Cooking time: 25 minutes

Servings: 4

INGREDIENTS

- ★ ☐ 2pounds baby beets, peeled and halved

- ★ ☐ 1cup heavy cream

- ★ ☐ 1teaspoon turmeric powder

- ★ ☐ A pinch of salt and black pepper

- ★ ☐ 2tablespoons olive oil

- ★ ☐ 2garlic cloves, minced

- ★ ☐ Juice of 1 lime

- ★ ☐ ½ teaspoon coriander, ground

DIRECTIONS

1. In a pan that fits your air fryer, mix the beet with the cream, turmeric and the other ingredients, toss, introduce the pan in the fryer and cook at 400 degrees F for 25 minutes.

2. Divide between plates and serve.

Nutrition:

Calories 135, Fat 3, Fiber 2, Carbs 4, Protein 6

Chard and Olives

Preparation time: 5 minutes

Cooking time: 20 minutes

Servings: 4

INGREDIENTS

- ★ ☐ 2 cups red chard, torn

- ★ ☐ 1 cup kalamata olives, pitted and halved

- ★ ☐ ½ cup tomato sauce

- ★ ☐ 1 teaspoon chili powder

- ★ ☐ 2 tablespoons olive oil

- ★ ☐ Salt and black pepper to the taste

DIRECTIONS

1. In a pan that fits the air fryer, combine the chard with the olives and the other ingredients and toss.

2. Put the pan in your air fryer, cook at 370 degrees F for 20 minutes, divide between plates and serve.

Nutrition:

Calories 154,

Fat 3,

Fiber 2,

Carbs 4, Protein 6

Coconut Mushrooms Mix

Preparation time: 5 minutes

Cooking time: 20 minutes

Servings: 4

INGREDIENTS

- ★ ☐ 1pound white mushrooms, halved

- ★ ☐ 1teaspoon sweet paprika

- ★ ☐ 1red onion, chopped

- ★ ☐ 1teaspoon rosemary, dried

- ★ ☐ Salt and black pepper to the taste

- ★ ☐ 2tablespoons olive oil

- ★ ☐ 1cup coconut milk

DIRECTIONS

1.In a pan that fits your air fryer, mix the mushrooms with the paprika and the other ingredients and toss.

2.Put the pan in the fryer, cook at 380 degrees F for 20 minutes, divide between plates and serve.

Nutrition:

Calories 162,

Fat 4,

Fiber 1, Carbs 3, Protein 5

Kale and Tomatoes

Preparation time: 5 minutes

Cooking time: 20 minutes

Servings: 4

INGREDIENTS:

★ ☐ 2cups baby kale

★ ☐ 1pound cherry tomatoes, halved

★ ☐ 1cup mild salsa

★ ☐ 2scallions, chopped

★ ☐ 1tablespoon olive oil

★ ☐ A pinch of salt and black pepper

★ ☐ 2tablespoons chives, chopped

DIRECTIONS

1.In a pan that fits the air fryer, combine the kale with the tomatoes and the other ingredients and toss.

2.Put the pan in the air fryer and cook at 380 degrees F for 20 minutes.

3.Divide between plates and serve.

Nutrition:

Calories 140,

Fat 3, Fiber 2, Carbs 3, Protein 5

Brussels Sprouts and Tomatoes

Preparation time: 5 minutes

Cooking time: 20 minutes

Servings: 4

INGREDIENTS

- ★ ☐ 1pound Brussels sprouts, trimmed

- ★ ☐ ½ pound cherry tomatoes, halved

- ★ ☐ 2tablespoons tomato paste

- ★ ☐ 1cup chicken stock

- ★ ☐ ½ teaspoon sweet paprika

- ★ ☐ 1tablespoon olive oil

- ★ ☐ Salt and black pepper to the taste

- ★ ☐ 1tablespoon chives, chopped

DIRECTIONS

1. In a pan that fits the air fryer, mix the sprouts with the tomatoes and the other ingredients and toss.

2. Put the pan in the air fryer and cook at 380 degrees F for 20 minutes.

3. Divide between plates and serve.

Nutrition:

Calories 170, Fat 5, Fiber 3, Carbs 4, Protein 7

Italian Tomatoes

Preparation time: 5 minutes

Cooking time: 20 minutes

Servings: 4

INGREDIENTS

★ ☐ 1 pound cherry tomatoes, halved

★ ☐ 1 teaspoon Italian seasoning

★ ☐ 1 tablespoon basil, chopped

★ ☐ Juice of 1 lime

★ ☐ A pinch of salt and black pepper

★ ☐ 4 garlic cloves, minced

★ ☐ 2 tablespoons olive oil

DIRECTIONS

1. In a pan that fits the air fryer, mix the tomatoes with the seasoning and the other ingredients, put the pan in the fryer and cook at 380 degrees F for 20 minutes.

2. Divide between plates and serve.

Nutrition::Calories 173, Fat 6, Fiber 2, Carbs 4, Protein 5

Salsa Zucchini

Preparation time: 5 minutes

Cooking time: 20 minutes

Servings: 4

INGREDIENTS

- ★ ☐ 1 pound zucchinis, roughly sliced

- ★ ☐ 1 cup mild salsa

- ★ ☐ 1 red onion, chopped

- ★ ☐ Salt and black pepper to the taste

- ★ ☐ 2 tablespoons lime juice

- ★ ☐ 2 tablespoons olive oil

- ★ ☐ 1 teaspoon coriander, ground

DIRECTIONS

1. In a pan that fits your air fryer, mix the zucchinis with the salsa and the other ingredients, toss, introduce in the fryer and cook at 390 degrees F for 20 minutes.

2. Divide the mix between plates and serve.

Nutrition:

Calories 150,

Fat 4,

Fiber 2, Carbs 4, Protein 5

Green Beans and Olives

Preparation time: 5 minutes

Cooking time: 20 minutes

Servings: 4

INGREDIENTS

- ★ ☐ 1pound green beans, trimmed and halved

- ★ ☐ 1cup black olives, pitted and halved

- ★ ☐ 1cup kalamata olives, pitted and halved

- ★ ☐ 1red onion, sliced

- ★ ☐ 2tablespoons balsamic vinegar

- ★ ☐ 1tablespoon olive oil

- ★ ☐ 3garlic cloves, minced

- ★ ☐ ½ cup tomato sauce

DIRECTIONS

1. In a pan that fits your air fryer, mix the green beans with the olives and the other ingredients, toss, put the pan in the fryer and cook at 350 degrees F for 20 minutes.

2. Divide the mix between plates and serve.

Nutrition: Calories 180, Fat 4, Fiber 3, Carbs 5, Protein 6

Spicy Avocado Mix

Preparation time: 5 minutes

Cooking time: 15 minutes

Servings: 4

INGREDIENTS:

★ ☐ 2small avocados, pitted, peeled and cut into wedges

★ ☐ 1tablespoon olive oil

★ ☐ Zest of 1 lime, grated

★ ☐ Juice of 1 lime

★ ☐ 1tablespoon avocado oil

★ ☐ A pinch of salt and black pepper

★ ☐ ½ teaspoon sweet paprika

DIRECTIONS

1.In a pan that fits the air fryer, mix the avocado with the lime juice and the other ingredients, put the pan in your air fryer and cook at 350 degrees F for 15 minutes.

2.Divide the mix between plates and serve.

Nutrition::

Calories 153,

Fat 3,

Fiber 3, Carbs 4, Protein 6

Spicy Black Beans

Preparation time: 5 minutes

Cooking time: 20 minutes

Servings: 4

INGREDIENTS

- ★ ☐ 2cups canned black beans, drained

- ★ ☐ 1tablespoon olive oil

- ★ ☐ 1teaspoon chili powder

- ★ ☐ 2red chilies, minced

- ★ ☐ Apinch of salt and black pepper

- ★ ☐ ¼ cup tomato sauce

DIRECTIONS

1. In a pan that fits the air fryer, mix the beans with the oil and the other ingredients, toss, put the pan in the air fryer and cook at 380 degrees F for 20minutes.

2. Divide between plates and serve.

Nutrition:

Calories 160,

Fat 4,

Fiber 3,

Carbs 5, Protein 4

Olives and Sweet Potatoes

Preparation time: 5 minutes

Cooking time: 25 minutes

Servings: 4

INGREDIENTS

- ★ ☐ 1pound sweet potatoes, peeled and cut into wedges

- ★ ☐ 1cup kalamata olives, pitted and halved

- ★ ☐ 1tablespoon olive oil

- ★ ☐ 2tablespoons balsamic vinegar

- ★ ☐ A bunch of cilantro, chopped

- ★ ☐ Salt and black pepper to the taste

- ★ ☐ 1tablespoon basil, chopped

DIRECTIONS

1. In a pan that fits the air fryer, combine the potatoes with the olives and the other ingredients and toss.

2. Put the pan in the air fryer and cook at 370 degrees F for 25 minutes.

3. Divide between plates and serve.

Nutrition:

Calories 132,

Fat 4, Fiber 2, Carbs 4, Protein 4

Spinach and Sprouts

Preparation time: 5 minutes

Cooking time: 20 minutes

Servings: 4

INGREDIENTS

☐ 1 pound Brussels sprouts, trimmed and halved

☐ ½ pound baby spinach

☐ 1 tablespoon olive oil

☐ Juice of 1 lime

☐ Salt and black pepper to the taste

☐ 1 tablespoon parsley, chopped

DIRECTIONS:

1. In the air fryer's pan, mix the sprouts with the spinach and the other ingredients, toss, put the pan in the air fryer and cook at 380 degrees F for 20 minutes.

2. Transfer to bowls and serve.

Nutrition:

Calories 140,

Fat 3,

Fiber 2,

Carbs 5, Protein 6

Cajun Tomatoes and Peppers

Preparation time: 4 minutes

Cooking time: 20 minutes

Servings: 4

INGREDIENTS

★ ☐ 1 tablespoon avocado oil

★ ☐ ½ pound mixed bell peppers, sliced

★ ☐ 1 pound cherry tomatoes, halved

★ ☐ 1 red onion, chopped

★ ☐ A pinch of salt and black pepper

★ ☐ 1 teaspoon sweet paprika

★ ☐ ½ tablespoon Cajun seasoning

DIRECTIONS

1. In a pan that fits the air fryer, combine the peppers with the tomatoes and the other ingredients, put the pan it in your air fryer and cook at 390 degrees F for 20 minutes.

2. Divide the mix between plates and serve.

Nutrition:

Calories 151, Fat 3, Fiber 2, Carbs 4, Protein 5

Lemon Tomatoes

Preparation time: 5 minutes

Cooking time: 20 minutes

Servings: 4

INGREDIENTS

- ★ ☐ 2pounds cherry tomatoes, halved

- ★ ☐ 1teaspoon sweet paprika

- ★ ☐ 1teaspoon coriander, ground

- ★ ☐ 2teaspoons lemon zest, grated

- ★ ☐ 2tablespoons olive oil

- ★ ☐ 2tablespoons lemon juice

- ★ ☐ A handful parsley, chopped

DIRECTIONS

1. In the air fryer's pan, mix the tomatoes with the paprika and the other ingredients, toss and cook at 370 degrees F for 20 minutes.

2. Divide between plates and serve.

Nutrition:

Calories 151,

Fat 2, Fiber 3, Carbs 5, Protein 5

Tomato and Green Beans

Preparation time: 5 minutes

Cooking time: 20 minutes

Servings: 4

INGREDIENTS

- ★ ☐ 1 pound cherry tomatoes, halved

- ★ ☐ ½ pound green beans, trimmed and halved

- ★ ☐ Juice of 1 lime

- ★ ☐ 1 teaspoon coriander, ground

- ★ ☐ 1 teaspoon sweet paprika

- ★ ☐ A pinch of salt and black pepper

- ★ ☐ 2 tablespoons olive oil

DIRECTIONS

1. In a pan that fits your air fryer, mix the tomatoes with the green beans and the other ingredients, toss, put the pan in the machine and cook at 380 degrees F for 20 minutes.

2. Divide between plates and serve.

Nutrition:

Calories 151,

Fat 3,

Fiber 2, Carbs 4, Protein 4

Cream Cheese Broccoli

Preparation Time: 5 min.

Cooking Time: 30 min.

Servings:: 2-3

Ingredients:

- ★ 1 tablespoon dry bread crumbs

- ★ 1/2 large onion, coarsely chopped

- ★ 1/2 (14 ounce) can evaporate milk

- ★ 1/2 cup sharp Cheddar cheese, cubed

- ★ 1 pound fresh broccoli, coarsely chopped

- ★ 2 tablespoons all-purpose flour

- ★ Salt to taste

- ★ 1 teaspoon butter

- ★ 1/4 cup

waDirections:

1.Place Instant Pot over kitchen platform. Place Air Fryer Lid on top. Press Air Fry, set the temperature to 375°F and set the timer to 5 minutes to preheat. Press "Start" and allow it to preheat for 5 minutes.

2.Take Air Fryer Basket, grease it with some cooking spray. In the basket, add milk and flour. Stir gently.

3.Place the basket in the inner pot of Instant Pot, close Air Fryer Lid on top.

4. Press the "Bake" setting. Set temperature to 360°F and set the timer to 5 minutes. Press "Start."

5. Open Air Fryer Lid after cooking time is over. Add broccoli and remaining milk.

6. Press the "Bake" setting. Set temperature to 360°F and set the timer to 5 minutes. Press "Start." Mix in cheese.

7. Combine crumbs and butter in a bowl. Add on top of the cheese.

8. Press the "Bake" setting. Set temperature to 360°F and set the timer to 20 minutes. Press "Start." Cook until the top is golden brown. Serve warm.

Nutrition:

Calories: 458

Fat: 19g

Saturated Fat: 5g

Trans Fat: 0g

Carbohydrates: 38g

Fiber: 7g

Sodium: 521mg

Protein: 23g

Mayonnaise Veggie Crumbs

Preparation Time: 5 min.

Cooking Time: 23 min.

Servings:: 4

Ingredients:

- ★ 1/2 zucchinis, sliced

- ★ 1/4 cup water

- ★ 1/4 cup mayonnaise

- ★ 1 tablespoon grated onion

- ★ 2 tablespoons butter, melted

- ★ 1/2 pound carrots, sliced

- ★ 1/4 teaspoon prepared horseradish

- ★ 1/4 teaspoon salt

- ★ 1/4 teaspoon ground black pepper

- ★ 1/4 cup Italian bread

crumbsDirections:

1.In a mixing bowl, combine well pepper, salt, horseradish, onion, mayonnaise, and water. In another bowl, combine crumbs and butter.

2.Place Instant Pot over kitchen platform. Place Air Fryer Lid on top. Press Air Fry, set the temperature to 375°F and set the timer to 5 minutes to preheat. Press "Start" and allow it to preheat for 5 minutes.

3. Take Air Fryer Basket, grease it with some cooking spray. In the basket, add carrots.

4. Place the basket in the inner pot of Instant Pot, close Air Fryer Lid on top.

5. Press the "Air Fry" setting. Set temperature to 360°F and set the timer to 8 minutes. Press "Start."

6. Open Air Fryer Lid after cooking time is over. Add zucchini.

7. Press the "Air Fry" setting. Set temperature to 360°F and set the timer to 5 minutes. Press "Start."

8. Add mayo mixture and toss well. Add crumb mixture on top.

9. Press the "Air Fry" setting. Set temperature to 390°F and set the timer to 10 minutes. Press "Start." Serve warm.

Nutrition:

Calories: 251

Fat: 16g

Saturated Fat: 5.5g

Trans Fat: 0g

Carbohydrates: 14g

Fiber: 3g

Sodium: 399mg

Protein: 3.5g

Air Fried Mushroom Vegetables

Preparation Time: 5 min.

Cooking Time: 15 min.

Servings:: 4

Ingredients:

- ★ 1 yellow squash, seeded and cut in circles

- ★ 1 zucchini, seeded and cut in circles

- ★ 1 teaspoon olive oil

- ★ 1 bunch asparagus spears, trimmed

- ★ 1 teaspoon basil powder

- ★ 1 teaspoon thyme

- ★ 1 cup button mushrooms, quartered

- ★ Black pepper (ground) and salt to

taste Directions:

1. In a mixing bowl, add seasoning and other ingredients. Combine to mix well with each other.

2. Place Instant Pot over kitchen platform. Place Air Fryer Lid on top. Press Air Fry, set the temperature to 375°F and set the timer to 5 minutes to preheat. Press "Start" and allow it to preheat for 5 minutes.

3. Take Air Fryer Basket, grease it with some cooking spray. In the basket, add a veggie mixture.

4. Place the basket in the inner pot of Instant Pot, close Air Fryer Lid on top.

5. Press the "Air Fry" setting. Set temperature to 375°F and set the timer to 15 minutes. Press "Start." Stir mixture halfway down.

6. Open Air Fryer Lid after cooking time is over. Serve warm.

Nutrition:

Calories: 46

Fat: 1.5g

Saturated Fat: 0g

Trans Fat: 0g

Carbohydrates: 6g

Fiber: 2.5g

Sodium: 301mg

Protein: 2g

Air Fried Broccoli Cauliflower

Preparation Time: 5-10 min.

Cooking Time: 15 min.

Servings:: 4-6

Ingredients:

- ★ 1 large yellow onion, cut into rings

- ★ 1 carrot, peeled and sliced

- ★ 2 small zucchinis, sliced

- ★ 1 yellow squash, seeded and sliced

- ★ 1 small head broccoli, cut into florets

- ★ ½ head cauliflower, cut into florets

- ★ Black pepper (ground) and salt to taste

- ★ ½ cup balsamic vinegar

- ★ 2 tablespoons

olive oil Directions:

1. In a mixing bowl, add seasoning and other ingredients. Combine to mix well with each other.

2. Place Instant Pot over kitchen platform. Place Air Fryer Lid on top. Press Air Fry, set the temperature to 375°F and set the timer to 5 minutes to preheat. Press "Start" and allow it to preheat for 5 minutes.

3. Take Air Fryer Basket, grease it with some cooking spray. In the basket, add a veggie mixture.

4. Place the basket in the inner pot of Instant Pot, close Air Fryer Lid on top.

5. Press the "Air Fry" setting. Set temperature to 350°F and set the timer to 15 minutes. Press "Start." Stir the mixture every 5 minutes. Note: Cook for 5 minutes if needed.

6. Open Air Fryer Lid after cooking time is over. Serve warm.

Nutrition: Calories: 133 Fat: 1.5g Saturated Fat: 0g Trans Fat: 0g Carbohydrates: 23.5g Fiber: 7g Sodium: 288mg Protein: 6g

Potato Cream Cheese

Preparation Time: 5-10 min.

Cooking Time: min.

Servings:: 4

Ingredients:

- ★ 4 tablespoon chives, chopped
- ★ 4 tablespoon Kalamata olives
- ★ 1 teaspoon onion powder
- ★ 4 medium russet potato, scrubbed and peeled
- ★ 4 teaspoon olive oil
- ★ 1/2 teaspoon salt
- ★ Butter, melted and cream cheese to taste

Directions:

1. Place Instant Pot over kitchen platform. Place Air Fryer Lid on top. Press Air Fry, set the temperature to 375°F and set the timer to 5 minutes to preheat. Press "Start" and allow it to preheat for 5 minutes.

2. Take Air Fryer Basket, grease it with some cooking spray. In the basket, add potatoes, olive oil, onion powder, salt, and butter; stir the mixture.

3. Place the basket in the inner pot of Instant Pot, close Air Fryer Lid on top.

4. Press the "Air Fry" setting. Set temperature to 400°F and set the timer to 40 minutes. Press "Start." Flip potatoes halfway down.

5. Open Air Fryer Lid after cooking time is over. Serve warm mixed with cream cheese, Kalamata olives, and chives.

Nutrition:

Calories: 133

Fat: 1.5g

Saturated Fat: 0g

Trans Fat: 0g

Carbohydrates: 23.5g

Fiber: 7g

Sodium: 288mg

Protein: 6g

SIDE DISH

Healthy Blueberry Muffins

Preparation Time: 10 min.

Cooking Time: 10 min.

Servings: 8-10

Ingredients:

- ★ ☐ teaspoons vanilla extract

- ★ ☐ 1 cup blueberries

- ★ ☐ ½ teaspoon salt

- ★ ☐ 1 cup yogurt

- ★ ☐ 1 ½ cups cake flour

- ★ ☐ ½ cup sugar

- ★ ☐ teaspoons baking powder

- ★ ☐ 1/3 cup vegetable oil

- ★ ☐ 1 egg

Directions:

1. Place your air fryer on a flat kitchen surface; plug it and turn it on. Set temperature to 355 degrees F and let it preheat for 4-5 minutes.

2. Take 10 muffin molds and gently coat them using a cooking oil or spray.

3. In a bowl of medium size, thoroughly mix the flour, sugar, baking powder and salt.

4. In a bowl of medium size, thoroughly mix the yogurt, oil, egg and vanilla extract. Mix both bowl mixtures. Add the chocolate chips.

5. Add the mixture into prepared muffin molds evenly.

6. Add the molds in the basket. Push the air-frying basket in the air fryer. Cook for 10 minutes.

7. Slide out the basket; serve warm!

Nutrition: Calories - 214   Fat – 8g   Carbohydrates – 32g   Fiber – 1g   Protein – 4g

Shrimp Bacon Bites

Preparation Time: 8-10 min.

Cooking Time: 8 min.

Servings: 8-10

Ingredients:

★ ☐ 1/2 teaspoon red pepper flakes, crushed

★ ☐ 1 tablespoon salt

★ ☐ 1 teaspoon chili powder

★ ☐ 1 ¼ pounds shrimp, peeled and deveined

★ ☐ 1 teaspoon paprika

★ ☐ 1/2 teaspoon black pepper, ground

★ ☐ 1 tablespoon shallot powder

★ ☐ 1/4 teaspoon cumin powder

★ ☐ 1 ¼ pounds thin bacon slices

Directions:

1. Place your air fryer on a flat kitchen surface; plug it and turn it on. Set temperature to 360 degrees F and let it preheat for 4-5 minutes.

2. Take out the air-frying basket and gently coat it using a cooking oil or spray.

3. In a bowl of medium size, thoroughly mix the shrimp and seasoning until they are coated well.

4. Now wrap a slice of bacon around the shrimps; secure them with a toothpick and refrigerate for 30 minutes.

5. Add the shrimps to the basket. Push the air-frying basket in the air fryer. Cook for 8 minutes.

6. Slide out the basket; serve with cocktail sticks or your choice of dip (optional).

Nutrition:

Calories – 374

Fat – 28.2g

Carbohydrates – 2g

Fiber – 0g

Protein – 34.3g

Beef Quinoa Meatballs

Preparation Time: 8-10 min.

Cooking Time: 15 min.

Servings: 5-6

Ingredients:

★ ☐ 1 cup quinoa, cooked

★ ☐ 1 beaten egg

★ ☐ 1/2 pound pork, ground

★ ☐ 1/2 pound beef, ground

★ ☐ scallions, chopped

★ ☐ 1/2 teaspoon onion powder

★ ☐ 1 ½ tablespoons Dijon mustard

★ ☐ 1 tablespoon sesame oil

★ ☐ tablespoons tamari sauce

★ ☐ 3/4 cup ketchup

★ ☐ 1 teaspoon ancho chili powder

★ ☐ 1/4 cup balsamic vinegar

★ ☐ tablespoons sugar

Directions:

1. In a bowl of medium size, thoroughly mix the ingredients and prepare small meatballs from it.

2. Place your air fryer on a flat kitchen surface; plug it and turn it on. Set temperature to 370 degrees F and let it preheat for 4-5 minutes.

3. Take out the air-frying basket and gently coat it using a cooking oil or spray.

4. Add the meatballs to the basket. Push the air-frying basket in the air fryer. Cook for 10 minutes.

5. Slide out the basket; shake and cook for 5 more minutes. Serve warm!

Nutrition: Calories - 292   Fat – 8.5g   Carbohydrates – 25g   Fiber – 6.4g   Protein – 26.3g

Buttery Apple Dumplings

Preparation Time: 8-10 min.

Cooking Time: 30 min.

Servings: 2-3

Ingredients:

★ 3 tablespoons raisins

★ 3 apples, smallest possible size, peeled and cored

★ 11 tablespoon brown sugar

★ 2 tablespoon butter, melted

★ 3 sheets puff pastry

1. Directions:

2. Place your air fryer on a flat kitchen surface; plug it and turn it on. Set temperature to 350 degrees F and let it preheat for 4-5 minutes.

3. Take out the air-frying basket and gently coat it using a cooking oil or spray.

4. Take the pastry sheets and place the apples in them; fill the cores with the sugar and raisin.

5. One by one, fold the pastries to form dumplings. Brush the butter all over the dumplings.

6. Add the dumplings in the basket. Push the air-frying basket in the air fryer. Cook for 25-30 minutes.

7. Slide out the basket; serve warm with your choice of dip!

Nutrition: Calories - 363   Fat – 20g   Carbohydrates – 23g   Fiber – 4g Protein – 5g

Spiced Squash Bites

Preparation Time: 8-10 min.

Cooking Time: 20 min.

Servings: 5-6

Ingredients:

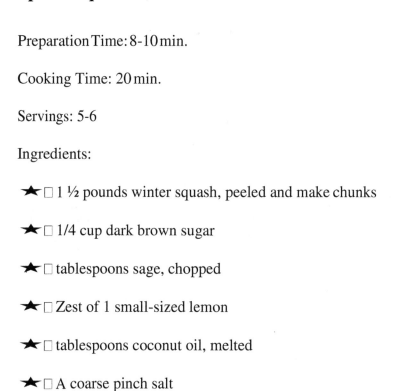

★ ☐ 1 ½ pounds winter squash, peeled and make chunks

★ ☐ 1/4 cup dark brown sugar

★ ☐ tablespoons sage, chopped

★ ☐ Zest of 1 small-sized lemon

★ ☐ tablespoons coconut oil, melted

★ ☐ A coarse pinch salt

★ ☐ A pinch pepper

★ ☐ 1/8 teaspoon allspice, ground

Directions:

1. Place your air fryer on a flat kitchen surface; plug it and turn it on. Set temperature to 350 degrees F and let it preheat for 4-5 minutes.

2. Take out the air-frying basket and gently coat it using a cooking oil or spray.

3. In a bowl of medium size, thoroughly mix the ingredients except for squash. Cover the squash chunks with the mixture.

4. Add the chunks to the basket. Push the air-frying basket in the air fryer. Cook for 10 minutes.

5. Increase temperature to 400 degrees F and cook for 8 more minutes. Serve warm!

Nutrition: Calories - 112   Fat – 4.6g   Carbohydrates – 18.6g   Fiber – 2g   Protein –1.7g

Yummy Potato Balls

Preparation Time: 8-10 min.

Cooking Time: 5 min.

Servings: 5-6

Ingredients:

★ ☐ 1/2 cup ham, chopped

★ ☐ 1/2 cup Colby cheese, shredded

★ ☐ ounces soft cheese

★ ☐ cups potatoes, mashed

★ ☐ 1 egg, slightly beaten

★ ☐ green onions, sliced

★ ☐ 1 cup seasoned breadcrumbs

★ ☐ ½ tablespoons canola oil

Directions:

1. Place your air fryer on a flat kitchen surface; plug it and turn it on. Set temperature to 390 degrees F and let it preheat for 4-5 minutes.

2. Take out the air-frying basket and gently coat it using a cooking oil or spray.

3. In a bowl of medium size, thoroughly mix the ingredients except for the breadcrumbs and canola oil.

4. Make small size balls from it.

5. Add the balls to the basket. Push the air-frying basket in the air fryer. Cook for 5 minutes.

6. Slide out the basket; serve warm!

Nutrition:

Calories – 368

Fat – 24.2g

Carbohydrates – 21g

Fiber – 4.1g

Protein – 17.6g

Banana Crunchy Chips

Preparation Time: 10-15 min.

Cooking Time: 15 min.

Servings: 3

Ingredients:

☐ pieces raw banana

☐ 1/2 teaspoon turmeric powder

☐ 1 teaspoon olive or your choice of oil

☐ ½ teaspoon chat masala or your favorite allspice mixture

☐ Salt as needed

Directions:

1. Place your air fryer on a flat kitchen surface; plug it and turn it on. Set temperature to 355 degrees F and let it preheat for 4-5 minutes.

2. Take out the air-frying basket and gently coat it using a cooking oil or spray.

3. In a bowl of medium size, thoroughly mix the turmeric powder, water, and salt. Take the bananas and make thin chips.

4. Cover the apple slices with the mixture and set aside for 10 minutes. Drain the liquid and dry the chips.

5. Add the chips to the basket. Push the air-frying basket in the air fryer. Cook for 15 minutes.

6. Slide out the basket; season the chips with chat masala and salt.

Nutrition: Calories - 340   Fat – 34g   Carbohydrates – 7g   Fiber – 4g   Protein – 5g

Savory Sausage Sides

Preparation Time: 5-8 min.

Cooking Time: 15 min.

Servings: 8-9

Ingredients:

★ ☐ ½ tsp. garlic puree

★ ☐ 3tbs. breadcrumbs

★ ☐ ½ onion, small size (peeled and diced)

★ ☐ to 4 oz. sausage meat

★ ☐ 1tsp. sage

★ ☐ Pepper and salt as required

Directions:

1. Place your air fryer on a flat kitchen surface; plug it and turn it on. Set temperature to 355 degrees F and let it preheat for 4-5 minutes.

2. Take out the air-frying basket and gently coat it using a cooking oil or spray.

3. In a bowl of medium size, thoroughly mix the ingredients and then prepare balls from it.

4. Add the meatballs to the basket. Push the air-frying basket in the air fryer. Cook for 14-15 minutes.

5. Slide out the basket; serve warm!

Nutrition:

Calories - 71   Fat – 1g   Carbohydrates – 12g   Fiber – 1g   Protein – 2g

Cheesy Mushrooms

Preparation Time: 8-10 min.

Cooking Time: 12 min.

Servings: 5-6

Ingredients:

- ★ □ tablespoons coriander, chopped

- ★ □ 1/3 teaspoon kosher salt

- ★ □ mushrooms, cut off the stems

- ★ □ 1/2 cup Gorgonzola cheese, grated

- ★ □ 1/2 teaspoon crushed red pepper flakes

- ★ □ 1/2 cup breadcrumbs

- ★ □ cloves garlic, pressed

- ★ □ 1 ½ tablespoons olive oil

- ★ □ 1/4 cup low-fat mayonnaise

- ★ □ 1 teaspoon prepared horseradish, drained

- ★ □ 1 tablespoon parsley, finely chopped

Directions:

1. Place your air fryer on a flat kitchen surface; plug it and turn it on. Set temperature to 380 degrees F and let it preheat for 4-5 minutes.

2. In a bowl of medium size, thoroughly mix the breadcrumbs, garlic, coriander, salt, red pepper, and olive oil.

3. Stuff the mushroom caps with the bread filling. Top with the cheese.

4. Add the mushrooms in the basket. Push the air-frying basket in the air fryer. Cook for 10-12 minutes.

5. Meanwhile, mix the mayonnaise, horseradish, and parsley. Serve with the warm mushrooms.

Nutrition: Calories - 212   Fat – 15.3g   Carbohydrates – 13.4g   Fiber – 4.2g   Protein – 7.4g

Corn & Carrot Fritters

Preparation Time: 8-10 min.

Cooking Time: 12 min.

Servings: 4-5

Ingredients:

★ ☐ ounces canned sweet corn kernels, drained

★ ☐ 1 teaspoon sea salt flakes

★ ☐ 1 tablespoon cilantro, chopped

★ ☐ 1 carrot, grated

★ ☐ 1 yellow onion, finely chopped

★ ☐ 1 medium-sized egg, whisked

★ ☐ 1/4 cup of self-rising flour

★ ☐ 1/3 teaspoon baking powder

★ ☐ tablespoons milk

★ ☐ 1 cup Parmesan cheese, grated

★ ☐ 1/3 teaspoon brown sugar

Directions:

1. Place your air fryer on a flat kitchen surface; plug it and turn it on. Set temperature to 350 degrees F and let it preheat for 4-5 minutes.

2. Press the carrot in the colander to remove excess liquid. Arrange the carrot between several sheets of kitchen towels and pat it dry.

3. Then, mix the carrots with the remaining ingredients in a big bowl. Make small balls from the mixture.

4. Gently flatten them with your hand. Spitz the balls with a nonstick cooking oil.

5. Add the in balls the basket.

6. Push the air-frying basket in the air fryer. Cook for 8-10 minutes.

7. Slide out the basket; serve warm!

Nutrition: Values:

Calories - 274

Fat – 8.3g

Carbohydrates – 38.8g

Fiber – 2.3g

Protein – 15.6g

Classic Bacon Shrimp Appetizer

Preparation Time: 10 min.

Cooking Time: 10 min.

Servings: 4-6

Ingredients:

★ ☐ ounces (around 16 slices) bacon, sliced

★ ☐ ounces (around 16 pieces) peeled shrimp, deveined

Directions:

1. Place your air fryer on a flat kitchen surface; plug it and turn it on. Set temperature to 390 degrees F and let it preheat for 4-5 minutes.

2. Now wrap the bacon over the shrimps. Refrigerate for about 15-20 minutes.

3. Add the shrimps to the basket. Push the air-frying basket in the air fryer. Cook for 6 minutes.

4. Slide out the basket; serve warm!

Nutrition:

Calories - 392

Fat – 25g

Carbohydrates – 8g

Fiber – 0g

Protein – 49g

Maple Bacon Tots

Preparation Time: 5-8 min.

Cooking Time: 18 min.

Smart Points: 5

Servings: 4-5

Ingredients:

- ★ ☐ tablespoons maple syrup

- ★ ☐ 1 cup Cheddar cheese, shredded

- ★ ☐ 24 frozen tater tots

- ★ ☐ slices precooked bacon

Directions:

1. Place your air fryer on a flat kitchen surface; plug it and turn it on. Set temperature to 355 degrees F and let it preheat for 4-5 minutes.

2. Add the tater tots in the air fryer basket. Cook for 9-10 minutes, shake the basket halfway through.

3. Meanwhile, make 1-inch pieces from bacon and shred the cheese. Take out the tots from the basket and arrange into a 6X6X2-inch pan.

4. Top with the bacon and maple syrup. Cook for 5 minutes or until the tots turn crisp. Top with the cheese; cook for 2 minutes and serve warm!

Nutrition: Calories – 372   Fat – 21.4g   Carbohydrates – 33.8g   Fiber – 2g   Protein – 13.4g

Mayo Tortellini Appetizer

Preparation Time: 10 min.

Cooking Time: 10 min.

Servings: 4-5

Ingredients:

★ ☐ ½ cup flour

★ ☐ ½ teaspoon dried oregano

★ ☐ 1 ½ cups breadcrumbs

★ ☐ ¾ cup mayonnaise

★ ☐ tablespoons mustard

★ ☐ 1 egg

★ ☐ tablespoons olive oil

★ ☐ cups cheese tortellini, frozen

Directions:

1. Place your air fryer on a flat kitchen surface; plug it and turn it on. Set temperature to 355 degrees F and let it preheat for 4-5 minutes.

2. In a bowl of medium size, thoroughly mix the mayonnaise and mustard. Set aside. In a bowl of medium size, thoroughly whisk the egg.

3. In another bowl, combine the flour and oregano. In another bowl, combine the breadcrumbs and olive oil.

4. Take the tortellini and add to the egg mixture, then into the flour, then into the egg again. Lastly, add the breadcrumbs to coat well.

5. Add the tortellini to the basket. Push the air-frying basket in the air fryer. Cook for 10 minutes until turn golden.

6. Slide out the basket; serve with the mayonnaise.

Nutrition: Calories - 542   Fat – 28.6g   Carbohydrates – 26.3g   Fiber – 3.6g   Protein – 18g

Eggs Spinach Side

Preparation Time: 5 min.

Cooking Time: 12 min.

Servings: 2-3

Ingredients:

★ ☐ 1 medium-sized tomato, chopped

★ ☐ 1 teaspoon lemon juice

★ ☐ 1/2 teaspoon coarse salt

★ ☐ tablespoons olive oil

★ ☐ eggs, whisked

★ ☐ ounces spinach, chopped

★ ☐ 1/2 teaspoon black pepper

★ ☐ 1/2 cup basil, roughly chopped

Directions:

1. Place your air fryer on a flat kitchen surface; plug it and turn it on. Set temperature to 280 degrees F and let it preheat for 4-5 minutes.

2. Take out the air-frying basket and gently coat it using the olive oil.

3. In a bowl of medium size, thoroughly mix the ingredients except for the basil leaves.

4. Add the mixture to the basket. Push the air-frying basket in the air fryer. Cook for 10-12 minutes.

5. Slide out the basket; top with basil and serve warm with sour cream!

Nutrition: Calories – 272   Fat – 23g   Carbohydrates – 5.4g   Fiber – 2g   Protein – 13.2g

Favorite Eggplant Caviar

Preparation Time: 20 min

Cooking Time: 20 min

Servings: 3

Ingredients

★ ☐ medium eggplants

★ ☐ ½ red onion

★ ☐ 1½ tbsp balsamic vinegar

★ ☐ 1 tbsp olive oil

Directions

1. Preheat the Air Fryer. Wash, then dry the eggplants.

2. Arrange them in a plate and cook them for 20 minutes at 360°F. Remove the eggplants from the oven and let cool down. Blend the onion in a blender.

3. Cut the eggplants in half, lengthwise, and empty their insides with a spoon. Put the inside of the eggplants in the mixer and process everything.

4. Add vinegar, olive oil and a little bit of salt, then blend again.

5. Serve cool with tomato sauce or ketchup.

Nutrition: Calories 287; Net Carbs 5.2g; Fat 7g; Protein 4g

Festive Cauli Croquettes

Preparation Time: 45 min

Cooking Time: 20 min

Servings: 4

Ingredients

★ ☐ cups cauli rice

★ ☐ 1 brown onion, chopped

★ ☐ garlic cloves, chopped

★ ☐ eggs, lightly beaten

★ ☐ ½ cup Parmesan cheese, grated

★ ☐ Salt and black pepper to taste

★ ☐ ½ cup pork rinds, crushed

★ ☐ 1 tsp dried mixed herbs

Directions

1. Combine cauli rice, onion, garlic, eggs, parmesan cheese, salt and pepper.

2. Shape into 10 croquettes. Spread the pork rinds onto a plate and coat each croquette in the pork rinds. Spray each croquette with oil.

3. Arrange the croquettes in the air fryer and cook for 16 minutes at 380°F, turning once halfway through cooking. They should be golden and crispy.

Nutrition: Calories 287; Net Carbs 5.2g; Fat 7g; Protein 4g

Orzo Salad

Preparation time: 10 minutes

Cooking Time: 10 minutes

Servings:: 6

Ingredients

- ★ 3 tsp red wine vinegar
- ★ 3 tsp olive oil
- ★ ½ tsp dried oregano
- ★ ½ tsp kosher salt
- ★ ¼ tsp freshly ground pepper
- ★ 1 jar marinated artichoke hearts
- ★ 1 jar roasted red pepper coarsely chopped
- ★ ½ large English cucumber diced
- ★ 1 cup pitted kalamata olives
- ★ ½ cup freshly chopped parsley
- ★ 6 ounces feta

cheese Directions:

1. Bring a large pot of salted water to boil. Whisk oregano, vinegar, oil, salt and a few grinds of black pepper and set them aside.

2. Add the orzo into the water and cool them for 10 minutes. drain and run briefly through cold water and allow them to cool.

3. Add peppers, cucumbers, artichoke hearts, red onions, and olives in a dressing bowl. Toss them thoroughly to allow them to combine them. add parsley and feta and toss them again. Allow it to sit for 20 minutes before stirring them from time to time to allow the flavors to blend well. Taste and season, it to your liking.

Nutrition: Calories 305.8 Fat 17g, Carbohydrates 28.9g, Proteins 9.3 g

Fondant Potatoes

Preparation time: 10 minutes

Cooking Time: 45 minutes

Servings:: 6

Ingredients

- ★ 3 cloves garlic
- ★ 4 medium potatoes
- ★ 4 tsp unsalted butter
- ★ ½ tsp kosher salt
- ★ ½ tsp freshly ground pepper
- ★ ¾ cup low sodium vegetable broth
- ★ 4 sprigs fresh thyme

Directions:

1. Peel the russet potatoes, trim the ends, and cut each potato into half. You should have 8 flat potato rounds. Put the potatoes in a large bowl and cover them with cold water. Allow it to sit for 20 minutes at room temperature to allow excess starch to be removed. Heat the oven and prepare butter and garlic.

2. Arrange a rack in the middle of the oven and heat it to 350 degrees Fahrenheit. Lightly smash and peel the 3 garlic cloves. Cut 4 tsp unsalted butter into 8 pieces.

3. Drain the potatoes and rise it with cold water. Pat them dry with paper towels. season the potatoes with ½ tsp black pepper and ½ tsp of kosher salt.

4. Heat 2 tablespoons of canola oil in a large oven and then add your potatoes cut side down in a single layer. Put them inside the oven and cook until they are brown. You will see the panel indicating that TURN FOOD.

5. When your instant fryer indicates this message flip the potatoes using tongs and add butter, garlic and 4 sprigs thyme and allow them to cook for 3 minutes. Cook until the butter begins to foam, then add ¾ cup vegetable broth.

6. Bake your potatoes until they are fork tender and slightly browned on the sides. This should take around 30 minutes, garnish with thyme sprigs before serving them drizzled with juices from your oven pan.

Nutrition:

Calories 180.4,

Fat 9.6g,

Carbohydrates 20.5g,

Protein 3.0 g,

Sodium: 156.1 Mg

Leftover Mashed Potato Pancakes

Preparation time: 20 minutes

Cooking Time: 10 minutes

Servings: 3

Ingredients

1 large egg - 1-ounce parmesan cheese

2 tsp chopped fresh chives - 2 cups cold mashed potatoes

½ cup all-purpose flour - 2 tsp olive oil

Sour cream for serving

Directions:

1. Grate an ounce of parmesan cheese and place it in a large bowl. Chop fresh chives until you have 2 tsps. Add one large egg and beat them with a wooden spoon to combine. Divide the potato mixture into 8 portions. Here you will work with one at a time.

2. Shape each portion into a patty around 3 inches diameter then dredge both sides into ¼ cup all-purpose flour. Shake of the excess and place them in a large baking sheet.

3. Heat the remaining olive oil in a baking try and using a wide spatula transfer the patties and allow them to cook. Press START on the panel and allow the food to cook. When the panel indicates TURN FOOD, flip the patties and allow the other side to cook.

4. Serve them warm with sour cream.

Nutrition: Calories 299.2, Fat 15.2g, Carbohydrates 30.3g, Protein 10.3 g, Fiber 2.0g, Sodium: 582.9mg.

Classic Corn Bread Dressing

Preparation: 20 minutes

Cooking Time; 45 minutes

Servings:: 7

Ingredients

- ★ 2 cups diced white onion
- ★ 1 recipe whole grain corn bread
- ★ 1 ½ cups diced celery
- ★ 2 tsp parsley finely chopped
- ★ 2 tsp fresh sage leaves
- ★ ¼ cup flat leaf parsley
- ★ 3 tsp canola oil
- ★ 2 large eggs
- ★ 1 tsp freshly ground black pepper
- ★ Cooking spray

½ tsp kosher salt

Directions:

1. Arrange your rack in the middle and heat the oven to 360 degrees Fahrenheit. Meanwhile be preparing 2 cups white onions, 1 ½ cup celery, finely chopped fresh sage leaves and put them in the same bowl. Coarsely chop until you have a ¼ cup of parsley leaves.

2. Heat 3 tsp canola oil over medium heat until it shimmers. Add onion, celery and cook while stirring until they are tender, this should take around 10 minutes. Add sage, thyme, 1 tsp black pepper, ½ tsp kosher salt and cook until fragrant. Remove from the heat and let it cool slowly.

3. Coat a low ceramic baking dish with cooking oil. Crumble cornbread in a large bowl. Beat two eggs, add the eggs to an onion mixture, 2 ½ cups of chicken stock and stir well for them to combine well. Transfer the mixture into a baking dish.

4. Put your instant air fryer into baking mode and press start. Baking until the dressing is lightly browned this is about 45 minutes. You can cover with an aluminum foil to prevent the mixture from being too browned.

5. Allow it to cook for 10 minutes before serving it.

Nutrition:

Calories 260.6,

Fat 11 g,

Carbohydrates 31.2 g,

Proteins 9.2 g,

Sodium: 421.6g.

Roasted Brussels Sprouts with Ginger and Scallions

Preparation time: 10 minutes

Cooking Time: 25 minutes

Servings:: 4

Ingredients

- ★ 3 tsp olive oil

- ★ 10 medium scallions

- ★ 2 tsp peeled grated ginger

- ★ 1-pound Brussel sprouts

- ★ 1 tsp low sodium soy sauce

- ★ ½ tsp kosher salt

- ★ Freshly ground pepper

Directions:

1. Put your instant air fryer oven on and arrange a rack in the middle of the oven. Allow it to gain temperature until it attains 380 degrees Fahrenheit. When it is ready place a parchment paper or baking sheet in the oven tray and trim half of the 1-pound Brussel sprouts.

2. Trim your scallions and cut them into ½ inch pieces, peel and mince them until you have 2 tsp of ginger.

3. Place the brussels sprouts and scallions on the baking sheet. Season with ginger and 3 tsp of olive oil, 1 tsp of low sodium soy sauce, ½ tsp kosher salt and a generous grind of black pepper.

4. Arrange the Brussel sprouts in a single layer cut side facing down. Bake them for 15 minutes or until the panel display TURN FOOD, flip them and allow the other side to cook as well. Once cooked the air fryer will go on standby mode. Taste and season with more sauce if you need.

Nutrition:

Calories 168.2

Fat 10.6g,

Carbs 13.5g,

Proteins 4.7g,

Sodium: 310.4 Mg

Bagna Cauda Roasted Brussels Sprouts

Preparation time: 10 minutes

Cooking Time: 25 minutes

Servings:: 4

Ingredients

- ★   4 anchovies

- ★   8 cloves garlic

- ★   ¼ cup olive oil

- ★   8 tsp unsalted butter

- ★   ½ tsp kosher salt

- ★   1-pound Brussel sprouts

★ Freshly ground pepper

Directions:

1. Put your oven on and put on baking mode on. Allow it to attain temperature of 380 degrees Fahrenheit. Meanwhile peal and thinly slice your garlic cloves. Rinse and pat your anchovies with paper towels and mince them. Place the anchovies and garlic in a small pan and add 1 stick of unsalted butter and ¼ cup of olive oil and simmer the Brussel sprouts until they are almost ready.

2. Trim and have the Brussel sprouts, place them in a hot baking sheet. Season the remaining ½ tsp kosher salt, 3 tsp olive oil, a generous grind of black pepper and toss them to combine fully. Arrange the Brussel sprouts in a single layer, cut side down.

3. Bake them for 15 minutes or until the panel indicates TURN FOOD, flip them and allow them to cook on the other side as well.

4. Once done, transfer the Brussel sprouts to a serving bowl and add Bagna cauda before tossing them and serving them.

Nutrition:

Calories 499,

Fat 47.4g,

Carbohydrates 12.5 G,

Proteins 5.6g,

Sodium: 409.2mg

Indian-ish Baked Potatoes

Preparation time: 10 minutes

Cooking Time: 45 minutes

Servings:: 4

Ingredients

- ★ ¼ cup sour cream

- ★ 1-pound baby red potatoes

- ★ 2 tsp kosher salt

- ★ ½ small red onion finely diced

- ★ 4 tsp minced ginger

- ★ 2 small Indian chilies

- ★ 2 tsp chaat masala

- ★ 2 tsp chopped fresh

cilanto Directions:

1. Preheat your oven to 400 degrees Fahrenheit. Peel and wash or just wash your baby potatoes and put them in a baking tray. Turn the baking mode on the instant air fryer. Bake them for 45 minutes or until they are fork tender. Allow them to cook until you are satisfied with the level.

2. Without cutting all the way to the bottom part, slice each potato into 4 . Use your hands to pull apart and push the four to make something like a blooming flower.

3. Sprinkle a pinch of salt in each potato before adding a tablespoon of sour cream. Evenly divide the onions, ginger, green chilies and chaat masala among the potatoes. Add chopped cilantro and serve while hot.

Nutrition: Calories 128.3, Fat 3.1g, Carbs 22.3g, Proteins 2.8g, Sodium: 15.2mg

Maple-Roasted Delicata Squash with Bacon

Preparation time: 10 minutes

Cooking Time: 25 minutes

Servings:: 4

Ingredients

- ★ 2 slices thick cut bacon

- ★ 1 tsp olive oil

- ★ 2 medium Delicata squash

- ★ 1 tsp pure Marple syrup

- ★ Freshly ground black pepper

- ★ Kosher salt

- ★ Chopped parsley

leaves Directions:

1. Put your instant air fryer on bake mode and allow it to attain 375 degrees Fahrenheit.

2. Trim 2 medium Delicata squash, cutting each half lengthwise and scrapping of the seeds and pulp.

3. Slice into ¼ inch and placed them in a rimmed parchment paper or a baking sheet. Cut 2 slices of bacon and add them into the baking sheet.

4. Drizzle the bacon and squash with 1 tsp olive oil and 1 tsp maple syrup. Season it with salt and pepper then toss them before spreading into an even.

5. Bake them for some time until the air fryer indicates TURN FOOD, flip them and allow the other side to cook as well. Once it is well done garnish with chopped parsley if that is what you like.

Nutrition: Calories 205 Fat 9.4 G, Carbohydrates 26.5g, Proteins 3.6g, Sodium:103.3 g

Brussels Sprouts with Bacon

Preparation time: 10 minutes

Cooking Time: 25 minutes

Servings:: 4

Ingredients

- ★ ¼ cup olive oil
- ★ 2 pounds Brussel sprouts
- ★ ¼ tsp red pepper flakes
- ★ Freshly ground black pepper
- ★ 2 tsp freshly squeezed lemon
- ★ 4 sliced uncured bacon
- ★ ¼ cup freshly grated parmesan cheese

Directions:

1. Put your vortex air instant fryer to bake mode and allow it to gain temperature until 380 degrees Fahrenheit. Meanwhile remove outer leaves and any undesired items from the 2 pounds of Brussel sprouts before trimming the ends. Keep the tiny ones as a whole and trim the large ones.

2. Put your Brussels in a parchment paper or rimmed baking sheet. Add ¼ cup of olive oil and season it with ½ tsp salt, black pepper and ¼ tsp red pepper flakes. Toss them and arrange them in a single layer on a baking tray.

3. Bake until the sprouts are lightly brown or until the panel indicates TURN FOOD, bake them until they turn crispy or brown to your liking. Cook the grated cheese and bacon in a pan and allow the cheese to melt before flipping. Transfer to a paper towel lined plate and grate ¼ cup parmesan cheese.

4. Transfer your Brussel sprouts into a serving bowl and drizzle with 2 tablespoons of lemon juice and toss them to combine. Taste before seasoning with salt and pepper to your liking.

Nutrition:

Calories 241.4

Fat 17.0g,

Carbohydrates 14.5g,

Proteins 7.6g,

Sodium: 357.1 Mg

Garlic Parmesan Monkey Bread

Preparation time: 30 minutes

Cooking Time: 25 minutes

Servings:: 4

Ingredients

- ★ 4 tsp unsalted butter
- ★ 1-pound pizza dough
- ★ 2 tsp olive oil
- ★ 4 cloves garlic minced
- ★ ½ tsp dried basil
- ★ ½ tsp dried parsley flakes
- ★ ½ tsp dried oregano
- ★ ½ cup freshly grated parmesan cheese
- ★ Koshe

r sDirections:

1. Coat an 8X5 inch pan with cooking oil. Cut the pizza dough into 1-ounce pieces and form each piece into a ball.

2. Stir your butter, oil, basil, garlic, oregano, and salt in a bowl. Add the dough ball into the bowl and toss them until they are well coated. Stack the dough balls in a pan and make 2 layers of 8 dough balls on each end.

3. Pour the remaining butter mixture over the dough, cover with a plastic wrap and set it in a warm spot to allow rising.

4. Put your instant air fryer oven into baking mode and allow it to attain the right temperature of 350 degrees Fahrenheit.

5. Uncover and sprinkle them with parmesan. Put them in the oven and bake them until they are golden brown at the center. Once done the panel will indicate the same. Remove and cool them in a rack. Invert the place and serve warm.

Nutrition:

Calories 543.9,

Fats 27.5g,

Carbohydrates 58.7g,

Proteins 15.4g,

Sodium 893.3mg,

Fibers 3.2g

Grilled Crash Potatoes

Preparation time: 10 minutes

Cooking Time: 40 minutes

Servings:: 4

Ingredients

- ★   1 lemon halved
- ★   1 tsp kosher salt
- ★   1 ½ pounds red potatoes
- ★   3 tsp olive oil
- ★   ½ tsp freshly ground pepper
- ★   1 clove garlic minced
- ★   2 tsp mayonnaise
- ★   2 stalks celery
- ★   ½ thinly sliced shallot
- ★   Fresh chives and

parsleyDirections:

1.Put your potatoes and a tablespoon of salt in a large pan and add enough cold water to cover them. Bring them to boil over high heat and reduce the heat and simmer until the potatoes can be pierced with a knife.

2. Meanwhile heat your oven frill to 380 degrees Fahrenheit. Dry your potatoes and place a parchment paper on a baking pan. Toss the potatoes with ¼ tsp pepper, ¾ tsp salt. Transfer the potatoes into a baking sheet and use a potato masher to flatten the potatoes to an inch thick.

3. Clean your oven and put the potatoes on the oven and allow them to bake until they are golden brown. Once the appliance indicates turn food. Flip them and allow the other side to cook as well until they are crispy and golden brown.

4. Whisk garlic, mayonnaise, paprika and the remaining ¼ tsp pepper, ¼ tsp salt and 1 tsp lemon juice in a large bowl.

5. Arrange your potatoes, shallots, celery, and grilled lemons in halves in a serving plate. Drizzle the dressing on top and sprinkle some herbs. Serve while hot.

Nutrition:

Calories 187.5,

Fat 10.7g,

Carbohydrates 20.3g,

Proteins 2.5g,

Sodium: 354mg.

Avocado Salad

Preparation time: 10 minutes

Cooking Time: 25 minutes

Servings:: 4

Ingredients

- ★ ½ small red onion

- ★ 1-pint cherry tomatoes

- ★ 2 medium avocados

- ★ ½ medium English cucumber chopped

- ★ ¼ tsp kosher salt

- ★ 2 tsp olive oil

- ★ ¼ tsp freshly ground black

pepperDirections:

1.Place your tomatoes, avocado, onion, cucumber and herbs in a large bowl. Squeeze lemon juice over the top and drizzle some oil. Gently toss them to combine well. Add salt and pepper and toss them some more to gel perfectly.

Nutrition:

Calories 272.2, Fat 21.8g, Carbohydrates 15.7g, Proteins 3.3g Fiber 8.7g, Sodium: 130.9mg

APETIZERS

Air Fry Bacon

Preparation Time: 5 minutes

Cooking Time: 10 minutes

Serving:11

Ingredients:

★ ☐ 11 bacon slices

Directions:

1. Place half bacon slices in air fryer basket.

2. Cook at 400 F for 10 minutes.

3. Cook remaining half bacon slices using same steps.

4. Serve and enjoy.

Nutrition:

☐ Calories 103

☐ Fat 7.9 g

☐ Carbohydrates 0.3 g

☐ Sugar 0 g

☐ Protein 7 g

☐ Cholesterol 21 mg

Crunchy Bacon Bites

Preparation Time: 5 minutes

Cooking Time: 10 minutes

Serving:4

Ingredients:

★ ☐ 4 bacon strips, cut into small pieces

★ ☐ 1/2 cup pork rinds, crushed

★ ☐ 1/4 cup hot sauce

Directions:

1. Add bacon pieces in a bowl.

2. Add hot sauce and toss well.

3. Add crushed pork rinds and toss until bacon pieces are well coated.

4. Transfer bacon pieces in air fryer basket and cook at 350 F for 10 minutes.

5. Serve and enjoy.

Nutrition:

☐ Calories 112

☐ Fat 9.7 g

☐ Carbohydrates 0.3 g

☐ Sugar 0.2 g

☐ Protein 5.2 g ☐ Cholesterol 3 mg

Easy Jalapeno Poppers

Preparation Time: 10 minutes

Cooking Time: 13 minutes

Serving:5

Ingredients:

☐ 5 jalapeno peppers, slice in half and deseeded

☐ 2 tbsp salsa

☐ 4 oz goat cheese, crumbled

☐ 1/4 tsp chili powder

☐ 1/2 tsp garlic, minced

☐ Pepper

☐ Salt

Directions:

1. In a small bowl, mix together cheese, salsa, chili powder, garlic, pepper, and salt.

2. Spoon cheese mixture into each jalapeno halves and place in air fryer basket.

3. Cook jalapeno poppers at 350 F for 13 minutes.

4. Serve and enjoy.

Nutrition: ☐ Calories 111 ☐ Fat 8.3 g ☐ Carbohydrates 2.1 g ☐ Sugar 1.2 g ☐ Protein 7.3 g ☐ Cholesterol 24 mg

Perfect Crab Dip

Preparation Time: 5 minutes

Cooking Time: 7 minutes

Serving:4

Ingredients:

☐ 1 cup crabmeat

☐ 2 tbsp parsley, chopped

☐ 2 tbsp fresh lemon juice ☐ 2 tbsp hot sauce

☐ 1/2 cup green onion, sliced

☐ 2 cups cheese, grated

☐ 1/4 cup mayonnaise ☐ 1/4 tsp pepper ☐ 1/2 tsp salt

Directions:

1.In a 6-inch dish, mix together crabmeat, hot sauce, cheese, mayo, pepper, and salt.

2.Place dish in air fryer basket and cook dip at 400 F for 7 minutes.

3.Remove dish from air fryer.

4.Drizzle dip with lemon juice and garnish with parsley.

5.Serve and enjoy.

Nutrition:

☐ Calories 313 ☐ Fat 23.9 g ☐ Carbohydrates 8.8 g ☐ Sugar 3.1 g ☐ Protein 16.2 g☐ Cholesterol 67 mg

Spinach Dip

Preparation Time: 10 minutes

Cooking Time: 40 minutes

Serving: 8

Ingredients: ☐ 8 oz cream cheese, softened

★ ☐ 1/4 tsp garlic powder

★ ☐ 1/2 cup onion, minced

★ ☐ 1/3 cup water chestnuts, drained and chopped

★ ☐ 1 cup mayonnaise

★ ☐ 1 cup parmesan cheese, grated

★ ☐ 1 cup frozen spinach, thawed and squeeze out all liquid

★ ☐ 1/2 tsp pepper

Directions:

1. Spray air fryer baking dish with cooking spray.

2. Add all ingredients into the bowl and mix until well combined.

3. Transfer bowl mixture into the prepared baking dish and place dish in air fryer basket.

4. Cook at 300 F for 35-40 minutes. After 20 minutes of cooking stir dip.

5. Serve and enjoy.

Nutrition: ☐ Calories 220 ☐ Fat 20.5 g ☐ Carbohydrates 9.3 g ☐ Sugar 2.3 g ☐ Protein 3.8 g ☐ Cholesterol 41 mg

Italian Dip

Preparation Time: 10 minutes

Cooking Time: 12 minutes

Serving: 8

Ingredients:

- ★ ☐ 8 oz cream cheese, softened

- ★ ☐ 1 cup mozzarella cheese, shredded

- ★ ☐ 1/2 cup roasted red peppers

- ★ ☐ 1/3 cup basil pesto

- ★ ☐ 1/4 cup parmesan cheese, grated

Directions:

1. Add parmesan cheese and cream cheese into the food processor and process until smooth.

2. Transfer cheese mixture into the air fryer pan and spread evenly.

3. Pour basil pesto on top of cheese layer.

4. Sprinkle roasted pepper on top of basil pesto layer.

5. Sprinkle mozzarella cheese on top of pepper layer and place dish in air fryer basket.

6. Cook dip at 250 F for 12 minutes.

7. Serve and enjoy.

Nutrition: ☐ Calories 115 ☐ Fat 10.7 g ☐ Carbohydrates 1.6 g ☐ Sugar 0.6 g ☐ Protein 3.6 g ☐ Cholesterol 34 mg

Sweet Potato Tots

Preparation Time: 10 minutes

Cooking Time: 31 minutes

Serving: 24

Ingredients:

★ ☐ 2 sweet potatoes, peeled

★ ☐ 1/2 tsp cajun seasoning

★ ☐ Salt

Directions:

1. Add water in large pot and bring to boil. Add sweet potatoes in pot and boil for 15 minutes. Drain well.

2. Grated boil sweet potatoes into a large bowl using a grated.

3. Add cajun seasoning and salt in grated sweet potatoes and mix until well combined.

4. Spray air fryer basket with cooking spray.

5. Make small tot of sweet potato mixture and place in air fryer basket.

6. Cook at 400 F for 8 minutes. Turn tots to another side and cook for 8 minutes more.

7. Serve and enjoy.

Nutrition:

☐ Calories 15☐ Fat 0 g ☐ Carbohydrates 3.5 g ☐ Sugar 0.1 g ☐ Protein 0.2 g ☐ Cholesterol 0 mg

Stuffed Mushrooms

Preparation Time: 10 minutes

Cooking Time: 15 minutes

Serving: 24

Ingredients:

★ □ 24 mushrooms, caps and stems diced

★ □ 1 1/2 tbsp mozzarella cheese, shredded

★ □ 1/2 cup sour cream

★ □ 1 cup cheddar cheese, shredded

★ □ 2 bacon slices, diced

★ □ 1 small onion, diced

★ □ 1/2 onion, diced

★ □ 1/2 bell pepper, diced

Directions:

1. Add diced mushrooms stems, bacon, carrot, onion, and bell pepper in pan and heat over medium heat.

2. Cook vegetable mixture until softened, about 5 minutes.

3. Stir in sour cream and cheddar cheese and cook until cheese is melted, about 2 minutes.

4. Preheat the air fryer 350 F.

5. Stuff vegetable cheese mixture into the mushroom cap and place in air fryer basket. Sprinkle mozzarella cheese on top.

6. Cook mushrooms for 8 minutes or until cheese is melted.

7. Serve and enjoy.

Nutrition:

☐ Calories 97

☐ Fat 7.4 g

☐ Carbohydrates 1.5 g

☐ Sugar 0.6 g

☐ Protein 6.4 g

☐ Cholesterol 20 mg

Herb Zucchini Slices

Preparation Time: 10 minutes

Cooking Time: 15 minutes

Serving: 4

Ingredients:

★ ☐ 2 zucchinis, slice in half lengthwise and cut each half through middle

★ ☐ 1 tbsp olive oil

★ ☐ 4 tbsp parmesan cheese, grated

★ ☐ 2 tbsp almond flour

★ ☐ 1 tbsp parsley, chopped

★ ☐ Pepper

★ ☐ Salt

Directions:

1. Preheat the air fryer to 350 F.

2. In a bowl, mix together cheese, parsley, oil, almond flour, pepper, and salt.

3. Top zucchini pieces with cheese mixture and place in the air fryer basket.

4. Cook zucchini for 15 minutes at 350 F.

5. Serve and enjoy.

Nutrition:

☐ Calories 157

☐ Fat 11.4 g

☐ Carbohydrates 5.1 g

☐ Sugar 1.7 g

☐ Protein 11 g

☐ Cholesterol 20 mg

Ranch Kale Chips

Preparation Time: 5 minutes

Cooking Time: 5 minutes

Serve: 4

Ingredients:

★ ☐ 4 cups kale, stemmed

★ ☐ 1 tbsp Nutrition:al yeast flakes

★ ☐ 2 tsp ranch seasoning

★ ☐ 2 tbsp olive oil

★ ☐ 1/4 tsp salt

Directions:

1. Add all ingredients into the large mixing bowl and toss well.

2. Spray air fryer basket with cooking spray.

3. Add kale in air fryer basket and cook for 4-5 minutes at 370 F. Shake halfway through.

4. Serve and enjoy.

Nutrition:

☐ Calories 102

☐ Fat 7 g

☐ Carbohydrates 8 g

☐ Sugar 0 g ☐ Protein 3 g ☐ Cholesterol 0 mg

Curried Sweet Potato Fries

Preparation Time: 10 minutes

Cooking Time: 20 minutes

Serving: 3

Ingredients:

- ★ ☐ 2 small sweet potatoes, peel and cut into fries shape

- ★ ☐ 1/4 tsp coriander

- ★ ☐ 1/2 tsp curry powder

- ★ ☐ 2 tbsp olive oil

- ★ ☐ 1/4 tsp sea salt

Directions:

1. Add all ingredients into the large mixing bowl and toss well.

2. Spray air fryer basket with cooking spray.

3. Transfer sweet potato fries in the air fryer basket.

4. Cook for 20 minutes at 370 F. Shake halfway through.

5. Serve and enjoy.

Nutrition:

☐ Calories 118

☐ Fat 9 g

☐ Carbohydrates 9 g ☐ Sugar 2 g ☐ Protein 1 g ☐ Cholesterol 0 mg

Roasted Almonds

Preparation Time: 5 minutes

Cooking Time: 8 minutes

Serving: 8

Ingredients:

- ★ ☐ 2 cups almonds

- ★ ☐ 1/4 tsp pepper

- ★ ☐ 1 tsp paprika

- ★ ☐ 1 tbsp garlic powder

- ★ ☐ 1 tbsp soy sauce

Directions:

1. Add pepper, paprika, garlic powder, and soy sauce in a bowl and stir well.

2. Add almonds and stir to coat.

3. Spray air fryer basket with cooking spray.

4. Add almonds in air fryer basket and cook for 6-8 minutes at 320 F. Shake basket after every 2 minutes.

5. Serve and enjoy.

Nutrition:

☐ Calories 143 ☐ Fat 11.9 g ☐ Carbohydrates 6.2 g ☐ Sugar 1.3 g ☐ Protein 5.4 g ☐ Cholesterol 0 mg

Crispy Zucchini Fries

Preparation Time: 10 minutes

Cooking Time: 10 minutes

Serving: 4

Ingredients:☐ 2 medium zucchinis, cut into fries shape

★ ☐ 1/2 tsp garlic powder ☐ 1 tsp Italian seasoning

★ ☐ 1/2 cup parmesan cheese, grated

★ ☐ 1/2 cup almond flour

★ ☐ 1 egg, lightly beaten

★ ☐ Pepper

★ ☐ Salt

Directions:

1. Add egg in a bowl and whisk well.

2. In a shallow bowl, mix together almond flour, spices, parmesan cheese, pepper, and salt.

3. Spray air fryer basket with cooking spray.

4. Dip zucchini fries in egg then coat with almond flour mixture and place in the air fryer basket.

5. Cook zucchini fries for 10 minutes at 400 F.

6. Serve and enjoy.

Nutrition: ☐ Calories 147 ☐ Fat 10 g ☐ Carbohydrates 6 g ☐ Sugar 3 g ☐ Protein 9 g ☐ Cholesterol 49 mg

Cauliflower Dip

Preparation Time: 10 minutes

Cooking Time: 40 minutes

Serve: 10

Ingredients:

★ ☐ 1 cauliflower head, cut into florets

★ ☐ 1 1/2 cups parmesan cheese, shredded

★ ☐ 2 tbsp green onions, chopped

★ ☐ 2 garlic clove

★ ☐ 1 tsp Worcestershire sauce

★ ☐ 1/2 cup sour cream

★ ☐ 3/4 cup mayonnaise

★ ☐ 8 oz cream cheese, softened

★ ☐ 2 tbsp olive oil

Directions:

1. Toss cauliflower florets with olive oil.

2. Add cauliflower florets into the air fryer basket and cook at 390 F for 20-25 minutes. Shake basket halfway through.

3. Add cooked cauliflower, 1 cup parmesan cheese, green onion, garlic, Worcestershire sauce, sour cream, mayonnaise, and cream cheese into the food processor and process until smooth.

4. Transfer cauliflower mixture into the 7-inch dish and top with remaining parmesan cheese.

5. Place dish in air fryer basket and cook at 360 F for 10-15 minutes.

6. Serve and enjoy.

Nutrition:

☐ Calories 308

☐ Fat 29 g

☐ Carbohydrates 3 g

☐ Sugar 1 g

☐ Protein 7 g

☐ Cholesterol 51 mg

Buffalo Cauliflower Wings

Preparation Time: 10 minutes

Cooking Time: 14 minutes

Serving:4

Ingredients:

★ ☐ 1 cauliflower head, cut into florets

★ ☐ 1 tbsp butter, melted

★ ☐ 1/2 cup buffalo sauce

★ ☐ Pepper

★ ☐ Salt

Directions:

1. Spray air fryer basket with cooking spray.

2. In a bowl, mix together buffalo sauce, butter, pepper, and salt.

3. Add cauliflower florets into the air fryer basket and cook at 400 F for 7 minutes.

4. Transfer cauliflower florets into the buffalo sauce mixture and toss well.

5. Again, add cauliflower florets into the air fryer basket and cook for 7 minutes more at 400 F.

6. Serve and enjoy.

Nutrition:

☐ Calories 44

☐ Fat 3 g

☐ Carbohydrates 3.8 g

☐ Sugar 1.6 g

☐ Protein 1.3 g

☐ Cholesterol 8 mg

Spicy Kale Chips

Preparation Time: 5-10 min.

Cooking Time: 5 min.

Servings: 2-3

Ingredients: 1 bunch of Tuscan kale (stems removed and leaves cut into 2-inch pieces)

★   2 tablespoons olive oil 1/4 teaspoon crushed red pepper

★   1/4 teaspoon salt 1/4 teaspoon paprika

★   1/4 teaspoon garlic

powder Directions:

1. In a mixing bowl, add the olive oil, kale leaves, and spices. Combine the ingredients to mix well with each other.

2. Place Instant Pot Air Fryer Crisp over kitchen platform. Press Air Fry, set the temperature to 400°F and set the timer to 5 minutes to preheat. Press "Start" and allow it to preheat for 5 minutes.

3. In the inner pot, place the Air Fryer basket. In the basket, add the kale mixture.

4. Close the Crisp Lid and press the "Air Fry" setting. Set temperature to 390°F and set the timer to 5 minutes. Press "Start."

5. Halfway down, open the Crisp Lid, shake the basket and close the lid to continue cooking for the remaining time.

6. Open the Crisp Lid after cooking time is over. Season to taste and serve warm.

Nutrition: Calories: 82 Fat: 6g Saturated Fat: 1.5g Trans Fat: 0g Carbohydrates: 3g Fiber: 0.5g Sodium: 258mg Protein: 0.5g

Classic French Fries

Preparation Time: 5-10 min.

Cooking Time: 24 min.

Servings: 4

Ingredients:

1 pound sweet potatoes, cut into French Fries size

¼ teaspoon garlic powder

Salt to taste

Olive oil

Directions:

1. In a mixing bowl, add the olive oil, potatoes, salt, and garlic powder. Combine the ingredients to mix well with each other.

2. Place Instant Pot Air Fryer Crisp over kitchen platform. Press Air Fry, set the temperature to 400°F and set the timer to 5 minutes to preheat. Press "Start" and allow it to preheat for 5 minutes.

3. In the inner pot, place the Air Fryer basket. In the basket, add the potato mixture.

4. Close the Crisp Lid and press the "Air Fry" setting. Set temperature to 380°F and set the timer to 18-20 minutes. Press "Start."

5. Halfway down, open the Crisp Lid, shake the basket and close the lid to continue cooking for the remaining time.

6. Open the Crisp Lid after cooking time is over. Season to taste and serve warm.

Nutrition:

Calories: 156

Fat: 4.5g

Saturated Fat: 1g

Trans Fat: 0g

Carbohydrates: 22g

Fiber: 3g

Sodium: 93mg

Protein: 3.5g

Crunchy Zucchini Chips

Preparation Time: 5 min.

Cooking Time: 12 min.

Servings: 4

Ingredients:

- ★ 1 medium zucchini, thinly sliced

- ★ 3/4 cup Parmesan cheese, grated

- ★ 1 cup Panko breadcrumbs

- ★ 1 large egg,

beaten Directions:

1. In a mixing bowl, add the Parmesan cheese and panko breadcrumbs. Combine the ingredients to mix well with each other.

2. In a mixing bowl, beat the eggs. Coat the zucchini slices with the eggs and then with the crumb mixture. Spray the slices with some cooking spray.

3. Place Instant Pot Air Fryer Crisp over kitchen platform. Press Air Fry, set the temperature to 400°F and set the timer to 5 minutes to preheat. Press "Start" and allow it to preheat for 5 minutes.

4. In the inner pot, place the Air Fryer basket. Line it with a parchment paper, add the zucchini slices.

5. Close the Crisp Lid and press the "Air Fry" setting. Set temperature to 350°F and set the timer to 10-12 minutes. Press "Start."

6. Halfway down, open the Crisp Lid, shake the basket and close the lid to continue cooking for the remaining time.

7. Open the Crisp Lid after cooking time is over. Serve warm.

Nutrition:

Calories:

Fat: g

Saturated Fat: g

Trans Fat: 0g

Carbohydrates: g

Fiber: g

Sodium: mg

Protein: g

Cauliflower Fritters

Preparation Time: 5-10 min.

Cooking Time: 8 min.

Servings: 6-8

Ingredients:

- ★ 1/3 cup shredded mozzarella cheese

- ★ 1/3 cup shredded sharp cheddar cheese

- ★ ½ cup chopped parsley

- ★ 1 cup Italian breadcrumbs

- ★ 3 chopped scallions

- ★ 1 head of cauliflower, cut into florets

- ★ 1 egg

- ★ 2 minced garlic

doeDirections:

1. Blend the florets into a blender to make the rice like structure. Add in a bowl. Mix in the pepper, salt, egg, cheeses, breadcrumbs, garlic, and scallions. Prepare 15 patties from the mixture. Coat them with some cooking spray.

2. Place Instant Pot Air Fryer Crisp over kitchen platform. Press Air Fry, set the temperature to 400°F and set the timer to 5 minutes to preheat. Press "Start" and allow it to preheat for 5 minutes.

3. In the inner pot, place the Air Fryer basket. In the basket, add the patties.

4. Close the Crisp Lid and press the "Air Fry" setting. Set temperature to 390°F and set the timer to 8 minutes. Press "Start."

5. Halfway down, open the Crisp Lid, shake the basket and close the lid to continue cooking for the remaining time.

6. Open the Crisp Lid after cooking time is over. Serve warm.

Nutrition:

Calories: 235

Fat: 19g

Saturated Fat: 8g

Trans Fat: 0g

Carbohydrates: 31g

Fiber: 5g

Sodium: 542mg

Protein: 6g

Lemon Potato Crisp

Preparation Time: 5-10 min.

Cooking Time: 18 min.

Servings: 4

Ingredients:

- ★ 1 teaspoon Cajun seasoning

- ★ ½ teaspoon ground black pepper

- ★ 1 teaspoon Italian seasoning

- ★ 1 teaspoon garlic powder

- ★ 1 pound baby potatoes, unpeeled and halved

- ★ 1 tablespoon virgin olive oil

- ★ 2 lemons, cut into wedges

- ★ 2 teaspoon kosher salt

- ★ ¼ cup finely chopped

parsley Directions:

1. In a mixing bowl, add the garlic powder, halved potatoes, Cajun seasoning, Italian seasoning, kosher salt, and potatoes. Combine the ingredients to mix well with each other.

2. Place Instant Pot Air Fryer Crisp over kitchen platform. Press Air Fry, set the temperature to 400°F and set the timer to 5 minutes to preheat. Press "Start" and allow it to preheat for 5 minutes.

3. In the inner pot, place the Air Fryer basket. In the basket, add the potatoes.

4. Close the Crisp Lid and press the "Air Fry" setting. Set temperature to 400°F and set the timer to 18 minutes. Press "Start."

5. Halfway down, open the Crisp Lid, shake the basket and close the lid to continue cooking for the remaining time.

6. Open the Crisp Lid after cooking time is over. Serve warm with lemon wedges and parsley on top.

Nutrition:

Calories: 159

Fat: 4g

Saturated Fat: 1g

Trans Fat: 0g

Carbohydrates: 22g

Fiber: 3.5g

Sodium: 619mg

Protein: 3.5g

Spiced Chickpeas

Preparation Time: 5-10 min.

Cooking Time: 20 min.

Servings: 4

Ingredients: 15.5 ounces canned chickpeas, drained and dried

★　　　　　　　　1 teaspoon salt　　¼ teaspoon cumin powder

★　　¼ teaspoon cayenne pepper

powder Directions:

1. Drain the canned chickpeas using a colander. Rinse and drain the water thoroughly. In a bowl, combine the spices.

2. Place Instant Pot Air Fryer Crisp over kitchen platform. Press Air Fry, set the temperature to 400°F and set the timer to 5 minutes to preheat. Press "Start" and allow it to preheat for 5 minutes.

3. In the inner pot, place the Air Fryer basket. In the basket, add the chickpeas.

4. Close the Crisp Lid and press the "Air Fry" setting. Set temperature to 390°F and set the timer to 20 minutes. Press "Start."

5. Halfway down, open the Crisp Lid, sprinkle half the seasoning mix, shake the basket and close the lid to continue cooking for the remaining time.

6. Open the Crisp Lid after cooking time is over. Sprinkle remaining seasoning and combine. Serve warm.

Nutrition: Calories: 186 Fat: 3.5g Saturated Fat: 0.5g Trans Fat: 0g Carbohydrates: 24g

Fiber: 6.5g Sodium: 789mg Protein: 8g

SNACKS

Zucchini Sauté

Preparation Time: 10 minutes

Cooking time: 20 minutes

Servings: 4

Ingredients:

- ★ 1 pound zucchinis, roughly cubed
- ★ 1 teaspoon sweet paprika
- ★ ½ cup heavy cream
- ★ 3 garlic cloves, minced
- ★ 1 tablespoon olive oil
- ★ Salt and black pepper to the taste
- ★ 2 tablespoons dill,

chopped Directions:

In your air fryer, combine the zucchinis with the paprika and the other Ingredients:, toss gently and cook at 370 degrees F for 20 minutes.

Divide between plates and serve as a side dish.

Nutrition: calories 109, fat 4, fiber 7, carbs 1, protein 2

Cumin Eggplant Mix

Preparation Time: 10 minutes

Cooking time: 20 minutes

Servings: 4

Ingredients:

- ★ 1 pound eggplant, roughly cubed

- ★ 1 cup cherry tomatoes, halved

- ★ 1 red onion, chopped

- ★ Salt and black pepper to the taste

- ★ 2 tablespoons olive oil

- ★ ½ teaspoon chili powder

- ★ ½ teaspoon cumin, ground

- ★ 1 tablespoon chives,

chopped Directions:

Heat up the air fryer with the oil at 350 degrees F, add the eggplants and the other Ingredients:, toss gently, and cook for 20 minutes.

Divide the mix between plates and serve as a side dish.

Nutrition:

calories 110,

fat 5, fiber 3, carbs 13, protein 9

Garlic Kale

Preparation Time: 10 minutes

Cooking time: 20 minutes

Servings: 4

Ingredients:

- ★ 1 pound kale leaves, torn

- ★ 1 tablespoon avocado oil

- ★ 1 teaspoon coriander, ground

- ★ 1 teaspoon basil, dried

- ★ 1 tablespoon balsamic vinegar

- ★ 4 garlic cloves, minced

- ★ Salt and black pepper to the

taste Directions:

In your air fryer, combine the kale with the oil and the other Ingredients:, toss well and cook them at 370 degrees F for 20 minutes.

Divide the mix between plates and serve as a side dish.

Nutrition:

calories 66,

fat 5,

fiber 8, carbs 11, protein 6

Green Beans Sauté

Preparation Time: 10 minutes

Cooking time: 20 minutes

Servings: 4

Ingredients:

- ★ 2 pounds green beans, trimmed and halved

- ★ Salt and black pepper to the taste

- ★ 1 tablespoon balsamic vinegar

- ★ 1 tablespoon dill, chopped

- ★ 2 tablespoons

olive oil Directions:

In your air fryer's basket, combine the green beans with the vinegar and the other Ingredients:, toss and cook at 350 degrees F for 20 minutes.

Divide between plates and serve as a side dish.

Nutrition:

calories 133,

fat 3,

fiber 8,

carbs 16,

protein 3

Herbed Tomatoes

Preparation Time: 10 minutes

Cooking time: 20 minutes

Servings: 4

Ingredients:

- ★ 1 pound tomatoes, cut into wedges

- ★ 2 tablespoons chives, chopped

- ★ 1 tablespoon oregano, chopped

- ★ 1 tablespoon balsamic vinegar

- ★ 1 teaspoon Italian seasoning

- ★ A pinch of salt and black pepper

- ★ 2 tablespoons olive

oil Directions:

In your air fryer's basket, combine the tomatoes with the chives, vinegar and the other Ingredients:, toss and cook at 360 degrees F for 20 minutes.

Divide everything between plates and serve as a side dish.

Nutrition:: calories 89, fat 7, fiber 9, carbs 4, protein 2

Coriander Potatoes

Preparation Time: 10 minutes

Cooking time: 25 minutes

Servings: 4

Ingredients:

- ★ 1 pound gold potatoes, peeled and cut into wedges

- ★ Salt and black pepper to the taste

- ★ 1 tablespoon tomato sauce

- ★ 2 tablespoons coriander, chopped

- ★ ½ teaspoon garlic powder

- ★ 1 teaspoon chili powder

- ★ 1 tablespoon

olive oil Directions:

In a bowl, combine the potatoes with the tomato sauce and the other Ingredients:, toss, and transfer to the air fryer's basket.

Cook at 370 degrees F for 25 minutes, divide between plates and serve as a side dish.

Nutrition: calories 210, fat 5, fiber 7, carbs 12, protein 5

Creamy Green Beans and Tomatoes

Preparation Time: 10 minutes

Cooking time: 20 minutes

Servings: 4

Ingredients:

- ★ 1 pound green beans, trimmed and halved

- ★ ½ pound cherry tomatoes, halved

- ★ 2 tablespoons olive oil

- ★ 1 teaspoon oregano, dried

- ★ 1 teaspoon basil, dried

- ★ Salt and black pepper to the taste

- ★ 1 cup heavy cream

- ★ ½ tablespoon cilantro,

chopped Directions:

In your air fryer's pan, combine the green beans with the tomatoes and the other Ingredients:, toss and cook at 360 degrees F for 20 minutes.

Divide the mix between plates and serve.

Nutrition: calories 174, fat 5, fiber 7, carbs 11, protein 4

Buttery Artichokes

Preparation Time: 10 minutes

Cooking time: 20 minutes

Servings: 4

Ingredients:

- ★ 4 artichokes, trimmed and halved

- ★ 3 garlic cloves, minced

- ★ 1 tablespoon olive oil

- ★ Salt and black pepper to the taste

- ★ 4 tablespoons butter, melted

- ★ ¼ teaspoon cumin, ground

- ★ 1 tablespoon lemon zest,

grated Directions:

In a bowl, combine the artichokes with the oil, garlic and the other Ingredients:, toss well and transfer them to the air fryer's basket.

Cook for 20 minutes at 370 degrees F, divide between plates and serve as a side dish.

Nutrition:

calories 214, fat 5, fiber 8, carbs 12, protein 5

Sweet Potato and Eggplant Mix

Preparation Time: 10 minutes

Cooking time: 20 minutes

Servings: 4

Ingredients:

- ★ 2 sweet potatoes, peeled and cut into medium wedges

- ★ 2 eggplants, roughly cubed

- ★ 1 tablespoon avocado oil

- ★ Juice of 1 lemon

- ★ 4 garlic cloves, minced

- ★ 1 teaspoon nutmeg, ground

- ★ Salt and black pepper to the taste

- ★ 1 tablespoon rosemary,

chopped Directions:

In your air fryer, combine the potatoes with the eggplants and the other Ingredients:, toss and cook at 370 degrees F for 20 minutes.

Divide the mix between plates and serve as a side dish.

Nutrition: calories 182, fat 6, fiber 3, carbs 11, protein 5

Peppers and Tomatoes Mix

Preparation Time: 5 minutes

Cooking time: 20 minutes

Servings: 4

Ingredients:

- ★ 1 tablespoon olive oil

- ★ 1 red onion, sliced

- ★ 1 pound cherry tomatoes, halved

- ★ 1 red bell pepper, cut into medium strips

- ★ 1 green bell pepper, cut in medium strips

- ★ 1 teaspoon chili powder

- ★ 1 teaspoon garam

masala Salt and black pepper to

the taste Directions:

In your air fryer, combine the tomatoes with the bell peppers and the other Ingredients:, toss and cook at 370 degrees F for 20 minutes.

Divide the mix between plates and serve as a side dish.

Nutrition:

calories 172,

fat 5, fiber 4, carbs 7, protein 4

Chives Carrots and Onions

Preparation Time: 5 minutes

Cooking time: 20 minutes

Servings: 4

Ingredients:

- ★ 1 pound baby carrots, peeled

- ★ 2 red onions, sliced

- ★ 1 tablespoon lime zest, grated

- ★ 1 tablespoon balsamic vinegar

- ★ 2 tablespoons chives,

chopped Directions:

In your air fryer's basket, combine the carrots with the onions and the other Ingredients:, toss and cook at 320 degrees F for 20 minutes.

Divide between plates and serve as a side dish.

Nutrition:

calories 132,

fat 4,

fiber 3,

carbs 11,

 protein 4

Cilantro Brussels Sprouts

Preparation Time: 5 minutes

Cooking time: 25 minutes

Servings: 4

Ingredients:

2 pounds Brussels sprouts, trimmed and halved

1 tablespoon olive oil

2 tablespoons maple syrup

1 tablespoon cilantro, chopped

1 tablespoon sweet paprika

A pinch of salt and black pepper

Directions:

In your air fryer's basket, combine the sprouts with the oil, maple syrup and the remaining Ingredients:, toss and cook at 360 degrees F for 25 minutes.

Divide between plates and serve as a side dish.

Nutrition:

calories 174,

 fat 5, f

iber 3,

 carbs 11, protein 4

Garlic Beets

Preparation Time: 10 minutes

Cooking time: 25 minutes

Servings: 4

Ingredients:

- 2 pounds beets, peeled and roughly cubed
- A pinch of salt and black pepper
- 1 teaspoon chili powder
- 4 garlic cloves, minced
- 1 tablespoon olive

oil Directions:

In your air fryer's basket, combine the beets with salt, pepper and the other Ingredients:, toss and cook at 370 degrees F for 25 minutes.

Divide the beets between plates and serve as a side dish.

Nutrition:

calories 171,

fat 4,

fiber 2,

carbs 13,

protein 3

Ginger Mushrooms

Preparation Time: 10 minutes

Cooking time: 20 minutes

Servings: 4

Ingredients:

- ★ 2 tablespoons olive oil

- ★ 2 tablespoons balsamic vinegar

- ★ 2 pounds white mushrooms, halved

- ★ 1 tablespoon ginger, grated

- ★ A pinch of salt and black pepper

- ★ 1 teaspoon cumin,

ground Directions:

In your air fryer's basket, combine the mushrooms with the oil, vinegar and the other Ingredients:, toss and cook at 360 degrees F for 20 minutes.

Divide the mix between plates and serve.

Nutrition:

calories 182, fat 3, fiber 2, carbs 8, protein 4

Masala Potatoes

Preparation Time: 10 minutes

Cooking time: 20 minutes

Servings: 4

Ingredients:

- ★ 2 pounds gold potatoes, peeled and roughly cubed

- ★ 1 tablespoon olive oil

- ★ 1 teaspoon garlic powder

- ★ 1 teaspoon garam masala

- ★ Juice of 1 lime

- ★ A pinch of salt and black

pepper Directions:

In your air fryer's basket, combine the potatoes with the garam masala and the other Ingredients:, toss and cook at 370 degrees F for 20 minutes.

Divide the mix between plates and serve.

Nutrition:

calories 182,

fat 4,

fiber 7,

carbs 12,

protein 4

Mixed Veggie Chips

Preparation Time: 20 minutes;

Cooking Time: 9 minutes;

Serving: 4

Ingredients:

- ★ 1 zucchini

- ★ 1 sweet potato peeled

- ★ 1/2 tsp pepper

- ★ 1 red beet, peeled

- ★ 1 large carrot

- ★ 1 tsp salt

- ★ 1 tsp Italian seasoning

- ★ A pinch cumin

powder Directions:

1. Preheat the air fryer in Dehydrate mode at 110 F for 2 to 3 minutes.

2. Meanwhile, use a mandolin slicer to thinly slice all the vegetables and transfer to a medium bowl. Season with salt, Italian seasoning, and cumin powder.

3. In batches, arrange some of the vegetables in a single layer on the cooking tray.

4. When the device is ready, slide the cooking tray onto the top rack of the oven and close the oven

5. Set the timer to 7 or 9 minutes and press Start. Cook until the vegetables are crispy.

6. Transfer the vegetables to serving bowls when ready and make the remaining in the same manner. Enjoy.

Nutrition:

Calories 84,

Total Fat 0.15g,

Total Carbs 18.88g,

Fiber 2.7g,

Protein 2.25g,

Sugar 1.94g,

Sodium 652mg

Sweet Apple and Pear Chips

Preparation Time: 15 minutes;

Cooking Time: 7 minutes;

Serving: 4

Ingredients:

★ 6 Honeycrisp apples

★ 6 pears, peeled

Directions:

1. Preheat the air fryer in Dehydrate mode at 110 F for 2 to 3 minutes.

2. Meanwhile, use a mandolin slicer to thinly slice the apples and pears.

3. In batches, arrange some of the fruit slices in a single layer on the cooking tray.

4. When the device is ready, slide the cooking tray onto the top rack of the oven and close the oven

5. Set the timer to 7 minutes and press Start. Cook until the fruits are crispy.

6. Transfer the fruit chips to serving bowls when ready and make the remaining in the same manner.

Enjoy.

Nutrition:

Calories 142,

Total Fat 0.46g,

Total Carbs 37.7g,

Fiber 6.6g,

Protein 0.71g,

Sugar 28.36g,

Sodium 3mg

Cocoa Banana Chips

Preparation Time: 5 minutes;

Cooking Time: 7 minutes;

Serving: 4

Ingredients:

- ★ 5 large firm banana, peeled

- ★ ¼ tsp cocoa powder

- ★ A pinch of cinnamon

powder Directions:

1. Preheat the air fryer in Dehydrate mode at 110 F for 2 to 3 minutes.

2. Meanwhile, use a mandolin slicer to thinly slice the bananas, and coat well with the cocoa powder and the cinnamon powder.

3. In batches, arrange as many banana slices as possible in a single layer on the cooking tray.

4. When the device is ready, slide the cooking tray onto the top rack of the oven and close the oven

5. Set the timer to 7 minutes and press Start. Cook until the banana pieces are crispy.

6. Transfer the chips to serving bowls when ready and make the remaining in the same manner. Enjoy.

Nutrition:

Calories 152,

Total Fat 0.57g,

Total Carbs 38.89g, Fiber 4.4g, Protein 1.87g, Sugar 20.79g, Sodium 2mg

Coriander Roasted Chickpeas

Preparation Time: 10 minutes;

Cooking Time: 45 minutes;

Serving: 2

Ingredients:

- ★ 1 (15 oz) can chickpeas, drained
- ★ 1/4 tsp ground coriander
- ★ 1/4 tsp curry powder
- ★ 1/4 tsp garlic powder
- ★ 1/4 tsp ground cumin
- ★ 1/4 tsp paprika
- ★ 1/8 tsp salt
- ★ 1/4 tsp chili pepper powder
- ★ Olive oil for

spraying Directions:

1. Preheat the oven in Air Fryer mode at 375 F for 2 to 3 minutes.

2. In a medium bowl, mix the chickpeas with all the spices until well combined and pour into the rotisserie basket. Grease lightly with olive oil, shake the basket, and close the seal.

3. Fix the basket onto the lever in the oven and close the oven.

4. Set the timer to 35 or 45 minutes, press Start and cook until the chickpeas are golden brown.

5. After, open the oven, take out the basket using the rotisserie lift and transfer the snack into serving bowls.

6. Allow cooling and enjoy.

Nutrition: Calories 91, Total Fat 1.82g, Total Carbs 14.87g, Fiber 4.2g, Protein 4.61g, Sugar 2.71g, Sodium 234mg

Parmesan Zucchini Chips

Preparation Time: 15 minutes;

Cooking Time: 7 minutes;

Serving: 4

Ingredients:

3 medium zucchinis

Salt to taste

1 cup grated Parmesan cheese

Directions:

1. Preheat the oven in Air Fryer mode at 110 F for 2 to 3 minutes.

2. Meanwhile, use a mandolin slicer to thinly slice the zucchinis, season with salt, and coat well with the Parmesan cheese.

3. In batches, arrange as many zucchini pieces as possible in a single layer on the cooking tray.

4. When the device is ready, slide the cooking tray onto the top rack of the oven and close the oven.

5. Set the timer to 7 minutes and press Start. Cook until the cheese melts while turning the halfway.

6. Transfer the chips to serving bowls to cool and make the remaining.

7. Serve warm.

Nutrition: Calories 107, Total Fat 6.99g, Total Carbs 3.73g, Fiber 0.1g, Protein 7.33g, Sugar 0.02g, Sodium 451mg

Ranch Garlic Pretzels

Preparation Time: 10 minutes;

Cooking Time: 15 minutes;

Serving: 4

Ingredients:

- ★ 2 cups pretzels
- ★ ½ tsp garlic powder
- ★ 1 ½ tsp ranch dressing mix
- ★ 1 tbsp melted

butter Directions:

1. Preheat the oven in Air Fryer mode at 270 F for 2 to 3 minutes.

2. In a medium bowl, mix all the ingredients until well combined, pour into the rotisserie basket and close to seal.

3. Fix the basket onto the lever in the oven and close the oven.

4. Set the timer to 15 minutes, press Start and cook until the pretzels are lightly browner.

5. After, open the oven, take out the basket using the rotisserie lift and transfer the snack into serving bowls.

6. Allow cooling and enjoy.

Nutrition:

Calories 35,

Total Fat 3.72g,

Total Carbs 0.4g,

Fiber 0g,

 Protein 0.12g,

Sugar 0.1g,

Sodium 40mg

Herby Sweet Potato Chips

Preparation Time: 12 minutes;

Cooking Time: 7 minutes;

Serving: 4

Ingredients:

★ 2 medium sweet potatoes, peeled

★ 1 tsp dried mixed herbs

★ 1 tbsp olive oil

Directions:

1. Preheat the oven in Air Fry mode at 375 F for 2 to 3 minutes.

2. Meanwhile, use a mandolin slicer to thinly slice the sweet potatoes, transfer to a medium bowl and mix well with the herbs and olive oil until well coated.

3. In batches, arrange as many sweet potato slices as possible in a single layer on the cooking tray.

4. When the device is ready, slide the cooking tray onto the top rack of the oven and close the oven.

5. Set the timer to 7 minutes and press Start. Cook until the sweet potatoes are crispy while turning halfway.

6. Transfer the chips to serving bowls when ready and make the remaining in the same manner. Enjoy.

Nutrition:

Calories 87,

Total Fat 3.48g,

Total Carbs 13.38g,

Fiber 1.9g,

Protein 1.03g,

Sugar 4.33g,

Sodium 20mg

Cumin Tortilla Chips with Guacamole

Preparation Time: 5 minutes;

Cooking Time: 15 minutes;

Serving: 4

Ingredients:

- ★ For the tortilla chips:
- ★ 12 corn tortillas
- ★ 2 tbsp olive oil
- ★ 1 tbsp cumin powder
- ★ 1 tbsp paprika powder
- ★ Salt and black pepper to

taste For the guacamole:

- ★ 1 large avocado, pitted and peeled
- ★ 1 small firm tomato, chopped
- ★ A pinch dried

parsley Directions:

1. Preheat the oven in Air Fry mode at 375 F for 2 to 3 minutes.

2. In a medium bowl, mix all the ingredients for the tortilla chips well and pour the mixture into the rotisserie basket. Close to seal.

3. Fix the basket onto the lever in the oven and close the oven.

4. Set the timer to 15 minutes, press Start and cook until the tortillas are golden brown.

5. After, open the oven, take out the basket using the rotisserie lift and transfer the chips to serving bowls.

6. Meanwhile, as the chips cooked, in a small bowl, mash the avocados and mix with the tomato and parsley until well combined.

7. Serve the tortilla chips with the guacamole.

Nutrition:

Calories 159,

Total Fat 14.74g,

Total Carbs 7.82g,

Fiber 4.6g,

Protein 1.94g,

Sugar 1.71g,

Sodium 9mg

Oven-Dried Strawberries

Preparation Time: 10 minutes;

Cooking Time: 7 minutes;

Serving: 4

Ingredients:

★ 1 lb. large strawberries

Directions:

1. Preheat the air fryer in Dehydrate mode at 110 F for 2 to 3 minutes.

2. Meanwhile, use a mandolin slicer to thinly slice the strawberries.

3. In batches, arrange some of the strawberry slices in a single layer on the cooking tray.

4. When the device is ready, slide the cooking tray onto the top rack of the oven and close the oven

5. Set the timer to 7 minutes and press Start. Cook until the fruits are crispy.

6. Transfer the fruit chips to serving bowls when ready and make the remaining in the same manner. Enjoy.

Nutrition:

Calories 36,

Total Fat 0.34g,

Total Carbs 8.71g, Fiber 2.3g, Protein 0.76g, Sugar 5.55g, Sodium 1mg

Chili Cheese Toasts

Preparation Time: 5 minutes;

Cooking Time: 8 minutes;

Serving: 4

Ingredients:

- ★ 6 slices sandwich bread
- ★ 4 tbsp butter
- ★ 1 cup grated cheddar cheese
- ★ 2 small fresh red chili, deseeded and minced
- ★ ½ tsp salt
- ★ 1 tsp garlic powder
- ★ 1 tsp red chili flakes
- ★ 1 tbsp chopped fresh

parsley Directions:

1. Preheat the oven in Broil mode at 375 F for 2 to 3 minutes.

2. Spread the butter on one side of each bread slices and lay on a clean, flat surface.

3. Divide the cheddar cheese on top and followed with the remaining ingredients.

4. Lay 3 pieces of the bread on the cooking tray, slide the tray onto the middle rack of the oven, and close the oven.

5. Set the timer for 3 to 4 minutes and press Start. Cook until the cheese melts and is golden brown on top.

6. Remove the first batch when ready and prepare the other three bread pieces.

7. Slice the into triangle halves and serve immediately.

Nutrition:

Calories 105,

Total Fat 11.53g,

Total Carbs 0.68g,

Fiber 0.1g,

Protein 0.29g,

Sugar 0.04g,

Sodium 388mg

DESSERTS

Tasty Banana Cake

Preparation time: 10 minutes

Cooking time: 30 minutes

Servings: 4

Ingredients: 1 tablespoon butter, soft

- 1 egg   1/3 cup brown sugar

- 2 tablespoons of honey

- 1 banana, peeled and mashed

- 1 cup white flour

- 1 teaspoon baking powder

- 1/2 teaspoon cinnamon powder

- Cooking spray

Directions:

1. Sprinkle a cooking spray on a cake pan and leave aside.

2. Combine butter and sugar, pineapple, tea, milk, cinnamon, baking powder and flour in a pot, and whisk

3. Pour this into a spray-filled cake pan, place it in your air fryer and cook for 30 minutes at 350 degrees F.

4. Left the cake to cool, chop and drink.

Nutrition: calories 270, fat 15, fiber 3, carbs 5, protein 9

Simple Cheesecake

Preparation time: 10 minutes

Cooking time: 15 minutes

Servings: 15

Ingredients:

- ★ ☐ 1 pound cream cheese

- ★ ☐ ½ teaspoon vanilla extract

- ★ ☐ 2 eggs

- ★ ☐ 4 tablespoons sugar

- ★ ☐ 1 cup graham crackers, crumbled

- ★ ☐ 2 tablespoons butter

Directions:

1. In a bowl, mix crackers with butter.

2. Press crackers mix on the bottom of a lined cake pan, introduce in your air fryer and boil for around 4 minutes at 350 degrees F.

3. Meanwhile, in a bowl, mix sugar with cream cheese, eggs and vanilla and whisk well.

4. Spread filling over crackers crust and cook your cheesecake in your air fryer at 310 degrees F for 15 minutes.

5. Slice the cake and serve.

Nutrition: calories 270, fat 15, fiber 3, carbs 5, protein 9

Bread Pudding

Preparation time: 10 minutes

Cooking time: 1 hour

Servings: 4

Ingredients:

- 6 crushed donuts

- 1 cup cherry

- 4 yolks

- 1 cup whipped cream and ½ cup

- Cup raisins

- Cup sugar

- Cup chocolate chips.

Directions:

1. Mix the cherries in a dish with the yolks of the egg and whipping cream, then mix well.

2. Mix the raisins and butter, chocolate chips and doughnuts in another dish, then swirl.

3. Combine the 2 mixtures, move everything to a greased pan which suits your air fryer and cook for 1 hour at 310 degrees F.

4. Once cooking, ice the pudding and eat. Enjoy!

Nutrition:

calories 302, fat 8, fiber 2, carbs 23, protein 10

Bread Dough and Amaretto Dessert

Preparation time: 10 minutes

Cooking time: 12 minutes

Servings: 12

Ingredients:

- ★ ☐ 1 pound bread dough

- ★ ☐ 1 cup sugar

- ★ ☐ ½ cup butter, melted

- ★ ☐ 1 cup heavy cream

- ★ ☐ 12 ounces chocolate chips

- ★ ☐ 2 tablespoons amaretto liqueur

Directions:

1. Roll dough, cut into 20 slices and then cut each slice in halves.

2. Brush dough pieces with butter, sprinkle sugar, place them in your air fryer's basket after you've brushed it some butter, cook them at 350 degrees F for 5 minutes, flip them, cook for 3 minutes more and transfer to a platter.

3. Heat up a pan with the heavy cream over medium heat, add chocolate chips and stir until they melt.

4. Add liqueur, stir again, transfer to a bowl and serve bread dippers with this sauce. Enjoy!

Nutrition: calories 200, fat 1, fiber 0, carbs 6, protein 6

Cinnamon Rolls and Cream Cheese Dip

Preparation time: 2 hours

Cooking time: 15 minutes

Servings: 8

Ingredients:

★ ☐ 1 pound bread dough

★ ☐ ¾ cup brown sugar

★ ☐ 1 and ½ tablespoons cinnamon, ground

★ ☐ ¼ cup butter, melted

★   For the cream cheese dip:

★ ☐ 2 tablespoons butter

★ ☐ 4 ounces cream cheese

★ ☐ 1 and ¼ cups sugar

★ ☐ ½ teaspoon vanilla

Directions:

1. Roll dough on a floured working surface, shape a rectangle and brush with ¼ cup butter.

2. In a bowl, mix cinnamon with sugar, stir, sprinkle this over dough, roll dough into a log, seal well and cut into 8 pieces.

3. Leave rolls to rise for 2 hours, place them in your air fryer's basket, cook at 350 degrees F for 5 minutes, flip them, cook for 4 minutes more and transfer to a platter.

4. In a bowl, mix cream cheese with butter, sugar and vanilla and whisk really well.

5. Serve your cinnamon rolls with this cream cheese dip.

Enjoy!

Nutrition: calories 200, fat 1, fiber 0, carbs 5, protein 6

Pumpkin Pie

Preparation time: 10 minutes

Cooking time: 15 minutes

Servings: 9

Ingredients:

- ★ ☐ 1 tablespoon sugar

- ★ ☐ 2 tablespoons flour

- ★ ☐ 1 tablespoon butter

- ★ ☐ 2 tablespoons water

For the pumpkin pie filling:

- ★ ☐ 3.5 ounces pumpkin flesh, chopped

- ★ ☐ 1 teaspoon mixed spice

- ★ ☐ 1 teaspoon nutmeg

- ★ ☐ 3 ounces water

- ★ ☐ 1 egg, whisked

★ ☐ 1 tablespoon sugar

Directions:

1. Put 3 ounces water in a pot, bring to a boil over medium high heat, add pumpkin, egg, 1 tablespoon sugar, spice and nutmeg, stir, boil for 20 minutes, take off heat and blend using an immersion blender.

2. In a bowl, mix flour with butter, 1 tablespoon sugar and 2 tablespoons water and knead your dough well.

3. Grease a pie pan that fits your air fryer with butter, press dough into the pan, fill with pumpkin pie filling, place in your air fryer's basket and cook at 360 degrees F for 15 minutes.

4. Slice and serve warm.

Enjoy!

Nutrition:

calories 200,

fat 5,

fiber 2,

carbs 5,

protein 6

Wrapped Pears

Preparation time: 10 minutes

Cooking time: 15 minutes

Servings: 4

Ingredients:

- 4 puff pastry sheets

- 14 oz vanilla custard

- half a pear

- 1 egg, whisk

- 1/2 teaspoon cinnamon powder

- 2 tablespoons sugar

Directions:

1. Place slices of puff pastry on a workbench, add a spoonful of vanilla custard to the center of each, and wrap half a pear over it.

2. Sprinkle eggs on the pear, sprinkle with sugar and cinnamon, place in an air fryer basket and cook at 320 degrees Fahrenheit for 15 minutes.

3. Divide parcels on plates and serve.

Enjoy!

Nutrition:

calories 200, fat 2, fiber 1, carbs 14, protein 3

Strawberry Donuts

Preparation time: 10 minutes

Cooking time: 15 minutes

Servings: 4

Ingredients:

★ ☐ 8 ounces flour

★ ☐ 1 tablespoon brown sugar

★ ☐ 1 tablespoon white sugar

★ ☐ 1 egg

★ ☐ 2 and ½ tablespoons butter

★ ☐ 4 ounces whole milk

★ ☐ 1 teaspoon baking powder

For the strawberry icing:

★ ☐ 2 tablespoons butter

★ ☐ 3.5 ounces icing sugar

★ ☐ ½ teaspoon pink coloring

★ ☐ ¼ cup strawberries, chopped

★ ☐ 1 tablespoon whipped cream

Directions:

1. In a bowl, mix butter, 1 tablespoon brown sugar, 1 tablespoon white sugar and flour and stir.

2. In a second bowl, mix egg with 1 and ½ tablespoons butter and milk and stir well.

3. Combine the 2 mixtures, stir, shape donuts from this mix, place them place in an air fryer basket and cook at 320 degrees Fahrenheit for 15 minutes.

4. Put 1 tablespoon butter, icing sugar, food coloring, whipped cream and strawberry puree and whisk well.

5. Arrange donuts on a platter and serve with strawberry icing on top.

Enjoy!

Nutrition:

calories 250,

fat 12,

fiber 1,

carbs 32,

protein 4

Air Fried Bananas

Preparation time: 10 minutes

Cooking time: 15 minutes

Servings: 4

Ingredients:

- 3 tablespoons butter

- 2 eggs

- 8 bananas, peeled and halved

- Cup cornflower

- 3 tablespoons cinnamon sugar

- 1 cup Panko

Directions:

Directions:

1. Heat the pan over medium high heat with butter, add panko, stir for 4 minutes, then transfer to a bowl.

2. Roll each with a mix of small flour, egg and panco, place in an air fryer basket, add cinnamon sugar, dust and cook at 280 degrees Fahrenheit for 10 minutes.

3. Please put out immediately. Enjoy!

Nutrition:

calories 164, fat 1, fiber 4, carbs 32, protein 4

Cocoa Cake

Preparation time: 10 minutes

Cooking time: 17 minutes

Servings: 6

Ingredients:

- ★ ☐ 3.5 ounces butter, melted

- ★ ☐ 3 eggs

- ★ ☐ 3 ounces sugar

- ★ ☐ 1 teaspoon cocoa powder

- ★ ☐ 3 ounces flour

- ★ ☐ ½ teaspoon lemon juice

Directions:

1. In a bowl, mix 1 tablespoon butter with cocoa powder and whisk.

2. In another bowl, mix the rest of the butter with sugar, eggs, flour and lemon juice, whisk well and pour half into a cake pan that fits your air fryer.

3. Add half of the cocoa mix, spread, add the rest of the butter layer and top with the rest of cocoa.

4. Put in your air fryer and boil at 360 degrees F for 17 minutes.

5. Cool cake down before slicing and serving.

Enjoy!

Nutrition: calories 340, fat 11, fiber 3, carbs 25, protein 5

Chocolate Cake

Preparation time: 10 minutes

Cooking time: 30 minutes

Servings: 12

Ingredients:

★ ☐ ¾ cup white flour

★ ☐ ¾ cup whole wheat flour

★ ☐ 1 teaspoon baking soda

★ ☐ ¾ teaspoon pumpkin pie spice

★ ☐ ¾ cup sugar

★ ☐ 1 banana, mashed

★ ☐ ½ teaspoon baking powder

★ ☐ 2 tablespoons canola oil

★ ☐ ½ cup Greek yogurt

★ ☐ 8 ounces canned pumpkin puree

★ ☐ Cooking spray

★ ☐ 1 egg

★ ☐ ½ teaspoon vanilla extract

★ ☐ 2/3 cup chocolate chips

Directions:

1. In a bowl, mix white flour with whole wheat flour, salt, baking soda and powder and pumpkin spice and stir.

2. In another bowl, mix sugar with oil, banana, yogurt, pumpkin puree, vanilla and egg and stir using a mixer.

3. Combine the 2 mixtures, add chocolate chips, stir, pour this into a greased Bundt pan that fits your air fryer.

4. Put in your air fryer and boil at 330 degrees F for 30 minutes.

5. Leave the cake to cool down, before cutting and serving it.

Enjoy!

Nutrition:

calories 232,

fat 7,

fiber 7,

carbs 29,

protein 4

Apple Bread

Preparation time: 10 minutes

Cooking time: 40 minutes

Servings: 6

Ingredients:

- ★ ☐ 3 cups apples, cored and cubed

- ★ ☐ 1 cup sugar

- ★ ☐ 1 tablespoon vanilla

- ★ ☐ 2 eggs

- ★ ☐ 1 tablespoon apple pie spice

- ★ ☐ 2 cups white flour

- ★ ☐ 1 tablespoon baking powder

- ★ ☐ 1 stick butter

- ★ ☐ 1 cup water

Directions:

1. In a bowl mix egg with 1 butter stick, apple pie spice and sugar and stir using your mixer.

2. Add apples and stir again well.

3. In another bowl, mix baking powder with flour and stir.

4. Combine the 2 mixtures, stir and pour into a spring form pan.

5. Put spring form pan in your air fryer and cook at 320 degrees F for 40 minutes

6. Slice and serve.

Enjoy!

Nutrition::

calories 192,

fat 6,

fiber 7,

carbs 14,

protein 7

Banana Bread

Preparation time: 10 minutes

Cooking time: 40 minutes

Servings: 6

Ingredients:

★ ☐ ¾ cup sugar

★ ☐ 1/3 cup butter

★ ☐ 1 teaspoon vanilla extract

★ ☐ 1 egg

★ ☐ 2 bananas, mashed

★ ☐ 1 teaspoon baking powder

★ ☐ 1 and ½ cups flour

★ ☐ ½ teaspoons baking soda

★ ☐ 1/3 cup milk

★ ☐ 1 and ½ teaspoons cream of tartar

★ ☐ Cooking spray

Directions:

1. In a bowl, mix milk with cream of tartar, sugar, butter, egg, vanilla and bananas and stir everything.

2. In another bowl, mix flour with baking powder and baking soda.

3. Combine the 2 mixtures, stir well, pour this into a cake pan greased with some cooking spray, introduce in your air fryer and cook at 320 degrees F for 40 minutes.

4. Take bread out, leave aside to cool down, slice and serve it.

Enjoy!

Nutrition:

calories 292,

fat 7,

fiber 8,

carbs 28,

protein 4

Mini Lava Cake s

Preparation time: 10 minutes

Cooking time: 20 minutes

Servings: 3

Ingredients:

- ★ ☐ 1 egg

- ★ ☐ 4 tablespoons sugar

- ★ ☐ 2 tablespoons olive oil

- ★ ☐ 4 tablespoons milk

- ★ ☐ 4 tablespoons flour

- ★ ☐ 1 tablespoon cocoa powder

- ★ ☐ ½ teaspoon baking powder

- ★ ☐ ½ teaspoon orange zest

Directions:

1. In a bowl, mix egg with sugar, oil, milk, flour, salt, cocoa powder, baking powder and orange zest, stir very well and pour this into greased ramekins.

2. Add ramekins to your air fryer and cook at 320 degrees F for 20 minutes.

3. Serve lava cakes warm.

Enjoy!

Nutrition: calories 201, fat 7, fiber 8, carbs 23, protein 4

Crispy Apple s

Preparation time: 10 minutes

Cooking time: 10 minutes

Servings: 4

Ingredients: □ 2 teaspoons cinnamon powder

□ 5 apples, cored and cut into chunks

□ ½ teaspoon nutmeg powder

□ 1 tablespoon maple syrup

□ ½ cup water

□ 4 tablespoons butter

□ ¼ cup flour

□ ¾ cup old fashioned rolled oats

□ ¼ cup brown sugar

Directions:

1. Put the apples in a pan that fits your air fryer, add cinnamon, nutmeg, maple syrup and water.

2. In a bowl, mix butter with oats, sugar, salt and flour, stir, drop spoonfuls of this mix on top of apples, introduce in your air fryer and cook at 350 degrees F for 10 minutes.

3. Serve warm.

Enjoy!

Nutrition: calories 200, fat 6, fiber 8, carbs 29, protein 12

Conclusion

There you have it guys! If you thought that the craze of air frying was too good to be true, you can finally give it a try and experience it for yourself. This miracle device gives your food a texture of deep frying with just a tablespoon or two of oil. With this device in your kitchen, you don't have to wait for state fairs and fast food shops to enjoy your fried delicacy – considering this is a healthy food option.

If you had an air fryer and didn't know what to cook in it, now you do – with all the recipes to for your breakfast, lunch, dinner, and desserts.

What are you still waiting for? Start cooking in your air fryer and enjoy all the foods you thought were not healthy!

Enjoy!